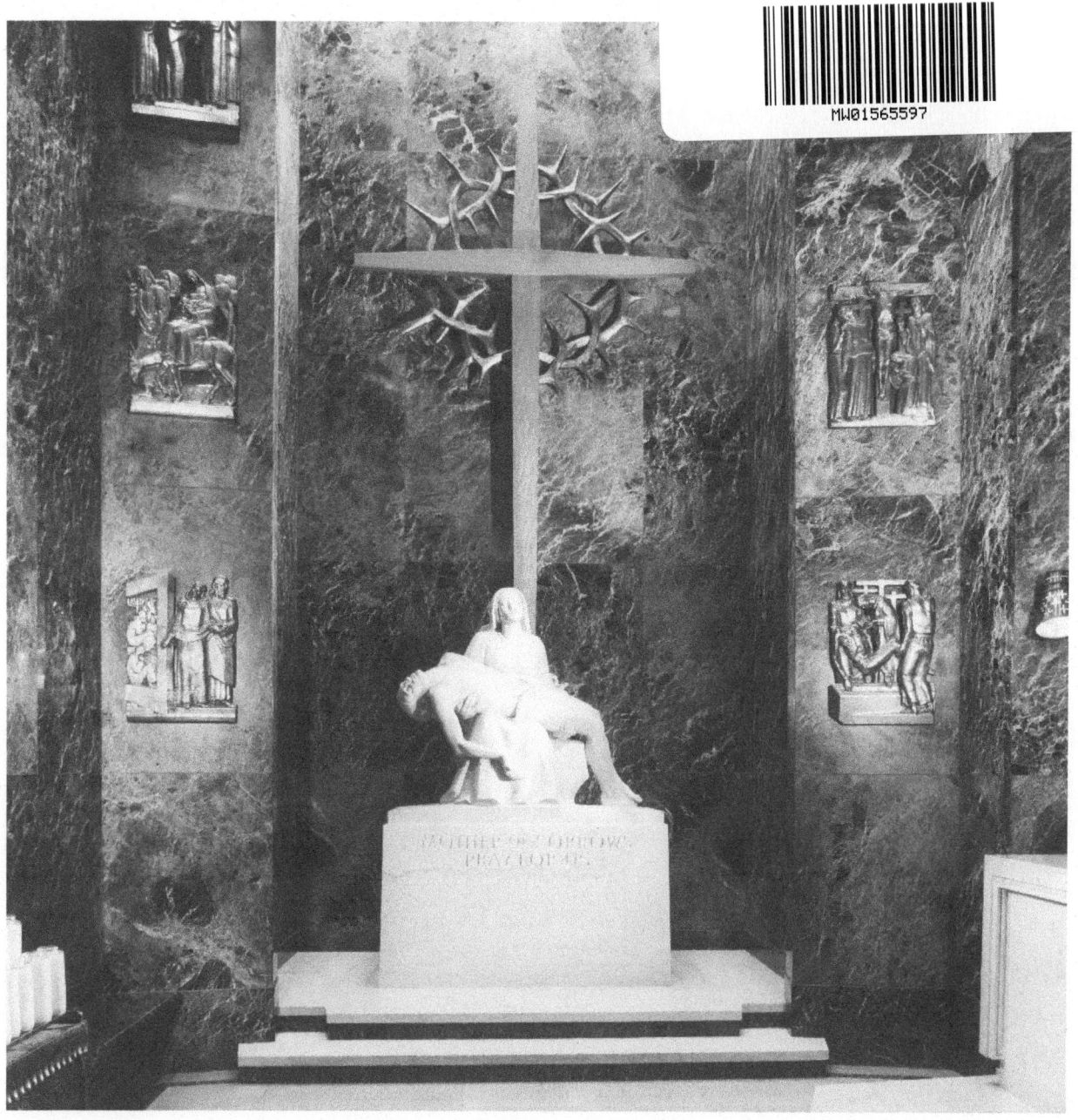

This book is dedicated to Mary, Our Mother of Sorrows.

The Chapel of Our Mother of Sorrows is located in the Great Upper Church of the Basilica at the National Shrine of the Immaculate Conception in Washington, D.C.

The Chapel features a life-size marble sculpture of the Pieta.

May your own devotion be strengthened by Mary's perseverance through every trial she faced. Following her example of unwavering faith, may we each draw near to Christ amid our suffering.

Alzheimer's Disease

ALZHEIMER'S DISEASE

A Caregiver's Guide
with Answers to
Questions

Robert H. Needham

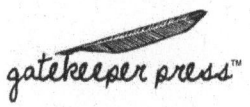

Columbus, Ohio

The views and opinions expressed in this book are solely those of the author and do not reflect the views or opinions of Gatekeeper Press. Gatekeeper Press is not to be held responsible for and expressly disclaims responsibility of the content herein.

Alzheimer's Disease: A Caregiver's Guide with Answers to Questions

Published by Gatekeeper Press
2167 Stringtown Rd., Suite 109
Columbus, OH 43123-2989
www.GatekeeperPress.com

Copyright © 2022 by Robert H. Needham

All rights reserved. Neither this book, nor any parts within it may be sold or reproduced in any form or by any electronic or mechanical means, including information storage and retrieval systems, without permission in writing from the author. The only exception is by a reviewer, who may quote short excerpts in a review.

The cover design work for this book are entirely the product of the author. Gatekeeper Press did not participate in and is not responsible for any aspect of these elements.

Library of Congress Control Number: 2022936001

ISBN (paperback): 9781662923685
eISBN: 9781662923692

Contents

SECTION ONE

Chapter 1

Understanding Dementia Diseases — 1

Types of Dementia Diseases — 1
Five Stages of Alzheimer's Disease — 3
Alzheimer's Facts — 5
Genetic Facts — 6
Testing and Medical Evaluation — 7
Diabetes Connection — 9

Chapter 2

Coping With Emotional and Behavioral Issues — 11

The Plight of Caregivers — 11
Caregivers Coping with Dementia Challenges — 12
Strategies for Managing a Patient's Emotional Challenges — 12
Strategies for Managing a Patient's Problematic Behavior — 14
Strategies for Managing the Caregiver's Emotional Challenges — 17
The Reluctant Caregiver — 23

SECTION TWO

Chapter 3

Caring Guidelines — 27

Breaking the News — 27
Taking the Car Keys — 27
Elder Mistreatment — 28
Dehydration — 30
Addressing Pain — 32
Hiring a nursing assistant (CNA) — 32
Medications — 33
Dentistry — 35

SECTION 3

Chapter 4
Responsible Planning 39
Financial and Legal Issues 39
Medicare and Medicaid Assistance 40
Advance Care Planning: Medical Issues to Consider 43

SECTION 4

Chapter 5
Corporate America and Alzheimer's 51
Impacting Corporate America 51
Caregivers: Rand Corporation 52

SECTION 5

Chapter 6
TIPS 53
Tips for the Caregiver 53

SECTION 6

Chapter 7
Resources 59
Helpful Resources for You and Your Family 59
References 63

APPENDIX A
Helpful Worksheets 65

APPENDIX B
The Story of Our Lady of Fatima 68

PREFACE

While writing this book, I read an article in the *Boston Globe* newspaper concerning a journalist describing his personal experience with Alzheimer's disease:

"In his powerful and poignant memoir, *On Pluto: Inside the Mind of Alzheimer's*, journalist Greg O'Brien provides readers with a gift-the opportunity to see his deeply personal experience with Alzheimer's disease through his eyes and those caregivers who most closely help him manage his condition: his family."

Mary Catherine McGeorge O'Brien notes in 'On Pluto,' when she began to care for her husband Greg, "I had no sense of where to turn for help, support, or even how to express the diagnosis with family, friends, or co-workers. I was lost and crept further inward. **There is no single handbook one can read to prepare; each journey is different, each course of the disease takes different meandering turns—no two are alike, the expert will tell you, an observation that is clearly numbing in so many ways.**"

At that point, I was certain that my book would provide people like Mary Catherine the handbook needed to manage the difficult journey of an Alzheimer's caregiver. Every 66 seconds someone in the US develops Alzheimer's disease with an estimate of nearly 500,000 new cases this year.

My life changed during a serendipitous encounter. While visiting a friend with dementia confined to a memory care facility, I found a new vocation. After filing the required paperwork, including an FBI background check, I became a full-time registered volunteer.

I spent three years in four different care centers in my community. I witnessed the many manifestations of the disease and the onerous requirements in caring for the afflicted. It was an opening of my emotional life. Perhaps, I was motivated by my Christian faith and a spontaneous desire to respond to the needs of others.

I was privileged to observe some insights into the frightful and sad disease of Alzheimer's. I noticed that as the progression of the disease unfolds, some very subtle, positive aspects of the patient are revealed. As the ego disappears, a genuine person sometimes emerges. They forget their need to impress, what clothes to wear, what to eat, or what to worry about. They are truly, "in the moment." The struggle just drops away.

Interestingly, all their worries and cares are simultaneously being transferred into the lives of their caregivers. Since up to 90% of Alzheimer patients receive their care at home from family members, I investigated how families without the resources for full-time help managed these challenges.

My research revealed many unsettling realities. The effect on the family can be overwhelming. In fact, gerontologists and psychologists often refer to the families of those with memory loss as the "invisible second patients." The physical, emotional, and financial toll on these caregivers is formidable, often leading to family conflict and early death.

The first need of a family that receives an Alzheimer's diagnosis is information. It's a struggle to gain some semblance of control, which is the goal of this book. The book will provide information about the disease, its progression, its manifestations, and techniques for managing behavioral and emotional challenges. The book will also guide the caregiver on the available medical coverage, financial and legal issues, and advanced care planning.

Hopefully, this book will become your companion on the long journey of caring for your loved one.

PURPOSE OF THE BOOK

Alzheimer's caregivers are dealing with the seventh leading cause of death in the United States affecting over 6.2 million people with no hope of recovery at this time. Alzheimer's disease is a progressive neurologic disorder that causes the brain to shrink (atrophy) and brain cells to die. It is the most common cause of dementia. Symptoms include a continuous decline in thinking, behavioral, and social skills that affects a person's ability to function independently.

When a family member is diagnosed with Alzheimer's or other dementias, the effect on the entire family can be overwhelming. The diagnosis can trigger a range of emotions, including anger, fear, frustration, and sadness. There also are many decisions to make about treatment, care, living arrangements, finances, and end-of-life care. As a result, family conflicts are common.

This book provides the basic information caregivers need to develop a plan to provide better care for their loved one. Many times, these caregivers are also seniors themselves and have the normal ailments that come with aging. Care becomes a twenty-four-hour, seven-days-a-week task that can last from five to fifteen years.

The purpose of this book is to address both the physical, spiritual, and personal needs of caregivers. While caregivers give care, they also need care as well.

On a physiological level, the book is brimming with disease definitions, typical disease progression, and suggestions on how to cope with behavioral and emotional issues. There is also a section on medical and financial planning issues, tips for facilitating daily management and traveling challenges, plus a guide on some of the most preeminent medical and research institutions for your personal research questions.

As the disease progresses, there are some medications that deal with various symptoms, but there are no cures and the demands on the caregiver become even more difficult and stressful. Over time the impact on the caregiver's health and mental state is significant. Caregivers aged 65 and under experience an increased death rate of 40% over the norm; if over age sixty-five, the death rate increases to *70%*.

On the spiritual level, we address the question asked by so many caregivers when overwhelmed by a task they did not ask for, were not trained for, and in their exhausted state, cry out "God Help Me!" Although the expectation of a miracle is possible, it seems what is really needed at that time is just some relief from a difficult task. It is like someone sitting too close to a roaring fire who just needs to be moved to a safer place.

This book is dedicated to Mary, Our Mother of Sorrows, due to Her example of a life of suffering and Her history of helping those in need. She is the ideal One to turn to when looking for relief from the stress and pain of caregiving. Unfortunately, many will ask, who is Mary, Our Mother of Sorrows?

Many non-religious have no idea of Her powers and many Christians, Biblical Literalist, teach little or nothing about the Mother of the Jesus they cherish. Therefore, generations of Christians have not heard of the many miracles God has performed in Her name. This book will be an introduction to Mary, Our Blessed Mother. For the first time some readers will learn of the peace and the many miracles attributed to Her under the names of: Our Lady of Lourdes, Our Lady of Fatima, Our Lady of Guadalupe, and many more.

Bishop Fulton J. Sheen proclaimed in 1952 that most famous marriage in history was at Cana, because Our Blessed Lord was present there. The Cana marriage is the only occasion in Sacred Scripture where Mary, the Mother of Jesus, is mentioned before Him.

It is a beautiful and a consoling thought that Our Blessed Lord, who came to teach, sacrifice, and urge us to take up our cross daily, should have begun His public life by assisting at a marriage feast. Sometimes these Eastern marriages lasted for seven days, but in the case of the poorer people, for only two. Whatever was the case, at Cana, at some period of the entertainment the wine suddenly ran out. This was very embarrassing because of the passionate devotion of the Eastern people to hospitality, and also because of the mortification it offered to the wedded pair.

One of the most amazing features of this marriage is that it was not the wine servant, whose business it was to service the wine, who noticed the shortage, but rather Our Blessed Mother. (She notes our needs before we ourselves feel them.) She made a very simple prayer to her Divine Son about the empty wine pots when she said: "They have no wine." Hidden in the words was not only a consciousness of the power of her Divine Son, but also an expression of her desire to remedy an awkward situation.

The answer of Our Blessed Lord was, "Woman what is that to me? My hour is not yet come."

In our own language, Our Lord was saying to His Blessed Mother: "My dear Mother, do you realize that you are asking me to proclaim my Divinity-to appear before the world as the Son of God, and to prove my Divinity by my works and my miracles? The moment that I do this, I begin the royal road to the Cross. When I am no longer known among men as the son of the carpenter, but as the Son of God, that will be my first step toward Calvary.

Once I undertake the salvation of mankind, you will not only be my mother, but you will also be the mother of everyone whom I redeem." The answer of Mary was one of complete cooperation in the Redemption of Our Blessed Lord, as she spoke for the last time in Sacred Scripture. Turning to the wine steward she said, "Whatsoever He shall say to you, that do ye." (John 2:5.)

But one thing is certain, no one will ever call on her without being heard, nor without being finally led to her Divine Son, Jesus Christ, for Whose Sake she alone exists, for Whose Sake she was made pure and for Whose Sake she was given to us.

On the Cross, with a gesture of His dust-filled eyes and His thorn-crowned head, He looks longingly at her and He says: "Behold thy son." Then, turning to John, He does not call him John; to do that would have been to address him as the son of Zebedee and no one else. But, in his anonymity, John stands for all of us. Our Lord thus says to His beloved disciple: "Son, behold thy mother."

Here is the answer, after all these years, to the mysterious words in the Gospel of the Incarnation which stated that Our Blessed Mother laid her "firstborn" in the manger. Did that mean that Our Blessed Mother was to have other children? It certainly did, but not according to the flesh. Our Divine Lord and Saviour Jesus Christ is the only Son of Our Blessed Mother by the flesh. But Our Lady was to have other children, not according to the flesh, but according to the spirit!

Who was Bishop Fulton J. Sheen?

Bishop Sheen was an American archbishop of the Roman Catholic Church known for his preaching and especially his work on radio and television. In the 1950s, his television show called "Life Is Worth Living" made him a household name. His timeless messages offer inspiring guidance, encouragement, peace of mind and spiritual comfort for millions of people. His one hour, Tuesday night TV show ran from 1951 until 1957, drawing as many as 30 million people a week. He wrote 73 books and numerous articles and columns. He dedicated his favorite book, "The World's First Love, Mary, the Mother of God," to "The Woman I Love." He went on to teach theology and philosophy at the Catholic University of America in Washington, D.C. He had a great love for the Blessed Mother, and even though he warned the world of godlessness and communism, he was a man of hope. He said that America, one way or the other, will be on its knees; either voluntarily or involuntarily.

Why not venerate The Blessed Virgin Mary?

None of the wonderful biblical writers and prophets we venerate in the Bible can compare to Mary.

Who was with Jesus at His conception?
Who was with Jesus at His birth?
Who raised Him as a child into manhood?
Who initiated His public life with at the wedding in Cana, as mentioned above?
Who was with Him at His death on the Cross?
Who did He give us as our Spiritual Mother with His few words from the Cross, as mentioned above?

Pentecost; Mary was with the eleven apostles at the birth of the Christian Church.

One of the most amazing stories Luke wrote about was the birth of the Savior. Elder Bruce R. McConkie (1915–85) of the Quorum of the Twelve Apostles says that Luke probably got his information about Jesus's birth from Mary herself because he did not know Jesus Christ personally. He became a follower after the Lord's death, when Paul taught him the gospel.

Perhaps neglecting The Blessed Mother of Jesus could be attributed to a diabolical influence.

Mary is God's aqueduct, through which He makes His mercies flow gently and abundantly. Therefore, She is the perfect resource to relieve the misery of millions of Alzheimer's caregivers. Her interventions on behalf of sufferers is legendary.

On the 13th of January 2004, Pope St. John Paul ll stated:

"If one wishes to rise quickly to holiness and perfection, there is no other way more pleasing to Christ than True Devotion to His Most Blessed Mother, the Immaculate Virgin Mary. Never was it known that anyone who fled to her protection implored her help, or sought her intercession was left unaided! She, the Mediator of all Graces, leads all her children to Christ."

SECTION ONE

CHAPTER 1

Understanding Dementia Diseases

Dementia is an overall term that describes a group of symptoms associated with a decline in memory or other thinking skills that reduce a person's ability to perform everyday activities. Alzheimer's accounts for up to 80% of these diseases. It starts slowly and gradually worsens over time. It can affect a person's mood, thinking, behavior, as well as their overall personality.

Types of Dementia Diseases

Alzheimer's

The most common early symptom is difficulty in remembering recent events. As the disease progresses, symptoms can include problems with language, disorientation, managing self-care and behavioral issues. As a person's condition declines, they often withdraw from family and society. Increasingly, bodily functions cease, eventually leading to death. The typical life expectancy following diagnosis is three to nine years.

Diffuse Lewy Body Disease

A degenerative brain disorder. Symptoms include cognitive impairments, fluctuation in level of alertness, reduced facial expression, shuffling gait, and tremors.

Normal Pressure Hydrocephalus

A disorder that obstructs the normal flow of cerebrospinal fluid. Symptoms include dementia, urinary incontinence, and difficulty walking.

Creutzfeldt-Jakob Disease (CJD)

A rare, fatal brain disorder caused by a transmissible infectious protein called a "prion." Symptoms include memory loss and lack of coordination. Causes involuntary movement and possible blindness.

Cerebral Amyloid Angiopathy (CAA)

Refers to protein deposits in blood vessels of the brain that can allow blood to leak out and cause bleeding strokes in the elderly. At the molecular level, it is also closely related to Alzheimer's disease through the protein amyloid-beta peptide. There is currently no effective prevention or treatment for CAA.

Progressive Supranuclear Palsy

An uncommon brain disorder that causes serious problems with walking, balance, and eye movements. The disorder results from deterioration of cells in areas of your brain that control body movement and thinking. It can worsen over time and can lead to pneumonia and swallowing problems.

Parkinson's Disease

A progressive disorder of the central nervous system. Characterized by tremors, stiffness in limbs and joints, speech impediments, and difficulty in starting physical movement.

Huntington's Disease

An inherited, degenerative brain disease which affects the mind and body. Characterized by intellectual decline, irregular and involuntary movements of the limbs or facial muscles, impaired judgment, and slurred speech.

Frontotemporal Dementia (Pick's disease)

Impacts personality and behavior and produces difficulty with speaking and understanding speech.

Five Stages of Alzheimer's Disease

Preclinical Stage

Changes in the brain known to be associated with Alzheimer's disease are happening during this stage, but the patient is not showing signs of disease. This stage can last for years or even decades. People in this stage are usually not diagnosed with Alzheimer's disease yet because they are functioning at a high level. However, there are now brain imaging tests that can detect deposits of a protein in the brain called amyloid. This protein interferes with the brain's communication system.

Moderate Stage

People in the moderate stage of Alzheimer's require assistance. People in this stage exhibit the following:

- Increased memory loss and confusion, often forgetting events or details about their own life
- Growing confusion about day of the week, season, and where they are
- Poor short-term memory
- Some difficulty recognizing friends and family
- Repeat stories or thoughts or events that are on their minds
- Difficulty with simple arithmetic
- May need help choosing proper attire and putting clothes in the right order
- Difficulty carrying out multi-step tasks
- May need some help with self-care, such as bathing, grooming, showering, and toileting
- Experience more changes in personality including being agitated and acting out
- May show delusional behavior, depression, apathy, or anxiety as the disease progresses
- May develop groundless suspicions about family, friends, and caregivers
- May begin to wander from their living area

Moderately Severe Stage

In this stage of Alzheimer's disease, the person manifests the following:

- May not consistently recognize his or her children, or spouse, or may confuse them with other family members
- May think strangers are family members
- Loses skills in dressing, bathing, and toileting
- Urinary incontinence, and later, fecal incontinence occurs

- Sleep is often disturbed
- Has significant confusion

Severe Stage

In this stage of Alzheimer's disease, the person displays the following:
- Has almost total memory loss
- Need helps with all basic activities of everyday living
- Is unaware of his or her surroundings
- Begins a decline in ability to sit up, walk, or eat without assistance
- Loses weight
- May have forgotten how to move his or her bowels or may be incontinent prior to reaching the toilet

Very Severe Stage

In this late stage of Alzheimer's disease, the person exhibits the following:
- Loses the ability to communicate; speech becomes limited to a few words and phrases.
- Forgets how to swallow. This can cause food and drink to enter the lungs and cause an infection.
- Loses ability to control bladder and bowel function
- Develops skin infection

Hospice care may be appropriate at this time for comfort. Common causes of death include pneumonia, malnutrition, dehydration, and other infections. Persons with Alzheimer's disease live on average four to eight years after diagnosis. Some patients can live as long as twenty years after diagnosis. The course of the disease varies.

Alzheimer's Facts

Throughout the world, over 50 million people are believed to suffer from Alzheimer's disease or other dementias. Every three seconds someone in the world develops dementia.

- More than 6 million Americans are living with Alzheimer's, and it's expected to increase by 14% annually.
- In 2050 it's estimated there will be as many as 16 million Americans living with Alzheimer's.
- It is estimated that nearly 500,000 new cases of Alzheimer's disease will be diagnosed this year in the United States. Every 66 seconds someone in the US develop Alzheimer's.
- One in three seniors die with some form of dementia.
- One in three Americans over the age of eighty-five are afflicted.
- Two of every three Alzheimer's patients are women.
- Black and Hispanic Americans are more likely to develop the disease than Caucasians.
- Thirty percent of Alzheimer's patients also have heart disease.
- Twenty-nine percent also have diabetes.
- It is the seventh leading cause of death across all ages, and sixth leading cause for those over age sixty-five.
- Alzheimer's deaths are currently underreported due to death certificates stating cause of death as choking, falling, heart failure, pneumonia, etc.
- A recent study found the Alzheimer's mortality rate to be five to six times higher than official estimates and may be responsible for more than 500,000 annual deaths in the US. If applied to the general population, these findings would make Alzheimer's the fourth (rather than seventh) leading cause of death behind heart disease, cancer, and COVID-19 (added last year).

Alzheimer's Bleak Future

- Between 2000 and 2017, deaths from heart disease decreased by 9% while deaths from Alzheimer's increased 145%.
- It kills more than breast cancer and prostate cancer combined.
- Alzheimer's and other dementia diseases are expected to cost the American healthcare system as much as $1.1 trillion in the future.
- Ten thousand Americans have turned sixty-five every day since January 2008. This trend will continue, and 10,000 more will turn sixty-five every day for the next fourteen years.
- Cases among Hispanics will increase seven times over today's estimates.
- Cases among Blacks will increase over four times.

Genetic Facts

Early-Onset Alzheimer's Disease

Early-onset Alzheimer's disease is rare, representing less than ten percent of all people with Alzheimer's. It typically occurs between a person's thirties and mid-sixties. Some cases are caused by an inherited change in one of three genes.

The three single-gene mutations associated with early-onset Alzheimer's disease are:
- Amyloid precursor protein (APP) on chromosome 21
- Presenilin 1 (PSEN1) on chromosome 14
- Presenilin 2 (PSEN2) on chromosome 1

A child whose biological mother or father carries a genetic mutation for one of these three genes has a 50/50 chance of inheriting that mutation. If the mutation is in fact inherited, the child has a very strong probability of developing early-onset Alzheimer's disease.

For other cases of early-onset Alzheimer's, research has shown that other genetic components are involved. Studies are ongoing to identify additional genetic risk variants.

Late-Onset Alzheimer's Disease

Most people with Alzheimer's have the late-onset form of the disease, in which symptoms become apparent in their mid-sixties and later.

Researchers have not found a specific gene that directly causes late-onset Alzheimer's disease. However, having a genetic variant of the apolipoprotein E (APOE) gene on chromosome 19 does increase a person's risk. The APOE gene is involved in making a protein that helps carry cholesterol and other types of fat in the bloodstream.

APOE ε4 is called a risk-factor gene because it increases a person's risk of developing the disease. However, inheriting an APOE ε4 allele does not mean that a person will definitely develop Alzheimer's. Some people with an APOE ε4 allele never get the disease, and others who develop Alzheimer's do not have any APOE ε4 alleles.

Recent research indicates that rare forms of the APOE allele may provide protection against Alzheimer's disease. More studies are needed to determine how these variations might delay disease onset or lower a person's risk.

For More Information About Alzheimer's Disease Genetics
NIA Alzheimer's and related Dementias Education and Referral (ADEAR) Center
800-438-4380 (toll-free)
adear@nia.nih.gov
www.nia.nih.gov/alzheimers

Testing and Medical Evaluation

To determine that Mild Cognitive Impairment (MCI) is due to Alzheimer's disease, a doctor must rule out other brain diseases or other causes--such as medications, depression, or major life changes that could account for cognitive decline.

If you have reason to believe your loved one may have a problem, a good option may be to take a simple online self-assessment cognitive test to determine if a problem may exist. Dementia Care Central on their website: dementiacarecentral.com offers an Alzheimer's/dementia online quick test for example, but there are quite a few to choose from.

From the Cleveland Clinic:

If you have a family history of Alzheimer's disease, you might sometimes feel a sense of worry about your own "senior slip-ups." If they seem to be happening more often as you get older, is that a sign that you're headed down the same path?

Advances in genetic testing have made it possible to get hints about your future health risks just by spitting in a cup or swabbing your cheek. But should you do it?

Some people feel empowered by learning about their genetic risk factors. For others, it can lead to more questions than it does answers.

From NIH: National Institute of Neurological Disorders and Stroke

A new blood testing technique could help researchers detect Alzheimer's disease prior to onset or in those showing early signs of dementia. The approach could be less invasive and costly than current brain imaging and spinal fluid tests, enabling earlier treatments and testing of novel approaches.

We don't yet completely understand the causes of late-onset AD, but they probably include genetic, environmental, and lifestyle factors. Although the risk of developing AD increases with age, AD and dementia symptoms are not a part of normal aging. There are also some forms of dementia that aren't related to brain diseases such as AD but are caused by systemic abnormalities such as metabolic syndrome, in which the combination of high blood pressure, high cholesterol, and diabetes causes confusion and memory loss.

Best advice for a definitive answer:

See a neurologist. A neurologist is a physician who specializes in disorders of the central and peripheral nervous system. They are often a key component in diagnosing dementia and Alzheimer's. A workup and full disclosure of your medical history by your family physician should be done prior to the appointment with the neurologist.

Diabetes Connection

Diabetes may increase your risk of Alzheimer's. Research suggests a connection between diabetes and Alzheimer's disease although those connections aren't yet fully understood. Not all studies confirm the connection, but many do suggest that people with diabetes, especially type 2 diabetes, are at higher risk of eventually developing Alzheimer's disease or other dementias.

According to Mayo Clinic studies:

"Diabetes can cause several complications, such as damage to your blood vessels. Diabetes is considered a risk factor for vascular dementia. This type of dementia occurs due to brain damage that is often caused by reduced or blocked blood flow to your brain.

"Many people with diabetes have brain changes that are hallmarks of both Alzheimer's disease and vascular dementia. Some researchers think that each condition fuels the damage caused by the other.

"Diabetes may also increase the risk of developing mild cognitive impairment (MCI) a condition in which people experience more thinking (cognitive) and memory problems than are usually present in normal aging. Some research indicates that diabetes may increase the risk of mild cognitive impairment worsening. MCI may precede or accompany Alzheimer's disease and other types of dementia."

CHAPTER 2

Coping With Emotional and Behavioral Issues

The Plight of Caregivers

Informal or unpaid caregiving has been associated with the following:
- Elevated levels of depression and anxiety
- Higher use of psychoactive medications
- Worse self-reported physical health
- Compromised immune function
- Increased risk of early death

Many families prefer to personally care for their loved one at home, or they cannot afford memory care facilities that can cost as much as $5,000 to $10,000 a month for 24/7 care. Eventually, home care takes its toll. Caregivers struggle to meet their loved ones needs and still carve out time for work, family time, hobbies, social engagements, and leisure time. Some become increasingly isolated. Home care can be a nightmare. Life becomes a day-to-day existence. As stated earlier, without proper support, the risk of dying for a caregiver aged sixty-five or younger increases by 40%. At age sixty-five or over, the risk increases to 70% compared to non-caregivers.

More Caregivers Will Be Needed

The CDC estimates that as the number of older Americans increases, so will the number of caregivers needed to provide care. The number of people sixty-five years old is expected to double between the years 2000 and 2030.

Ten thousand Americans have turned sixty-five every day since January 2008. This trend will continue, and 10,000 more will turn sixty-five every day for the next fourteen years. If you were born between 1946 and 1964, you are one of the 78 million Americans referred to as the baby boomers, the sandwich generation, and the silver tsunami. Millions are now sandwiched between retirement, caregiving, and raising children.

It is expected that there will be 71 million people aged sixty-five years old and older when all baby boomers are at least sixty-five years old in 2030.

Currently, there are seven potential family caregivers per adult. By 2030, there will be only four family caregivers available per adult.

Caregivers Coping with Dementia Challenges

The symptoms of Alzheimer's disease and other related dementias are typically memory-related, but mood and behavior swings also occur as the brain losses the ability to process information.

It can be devastating for a person's lifestyle, day-to-day routine, and social life to be interrupted and altered permanently by cognitive decline. Depression results. Loss of communication ability, access to memories, and general functionality result in a range of emotions including anger, frustration, and anxiety. Dementia also causes suspicion because situations become difficult to understand. The disease lowers a person's inhibitions in expressing emotions, resulting in outbursts or even spells of extreme laughter.

Behavior and emotions are distinct but often interrelated. Sleep disturbances may cause irritability, and hoarding is a result of anxiety. These emotional and behavioral changes are normal in the progression of dementia and can even be considered common and predictable. Remember that the two are related, and that addressing one challenge may help a multitude of others. Treating anxiety, for instance, may aid problems sleeping.

As the disease progresses you may have days when you get your loved one back as they were before, but you will likely have more days where they're easily angered, frustrated, or otherwise not themselves. None of their anger or frustration is your fault. They're not upset with you; they're upset with the disease that's robbed them of their ability to understand and feel comfortable in the world around them. Try to be patient and give yourself breaks. Taking care of yourself is as important as taking care of them.

Try not to take it personally; it is the disease talking and acting.

Strategies for Managing a Patient's Emotional Challenges

Although dementia is the direct result of damage to the brain, its manifestations often seem purely emotional. Often outside influences, like a change to living situations or routine, can exacerbate a patient's reaction to the disease. Outlined below are several common emotional problems and how best to handle them.

Anger:

Anger often arises from feelings of frustration or fear, and even embarrassment or a sense of humiliation. Losing control of their faculties, being unfamiliar with surroundings, or even momentarily unsure of the relationship with whoever is trying to assist them may cause your care-receiver to lash out. Harsh lights and sounds can also trigger a violent reaction.

Strategy:

Keep in mind that anger is the outward expression of something deeper. Try to determine what may be bothering your loved one. Is it too noisy; might there be too many people who appear to be strangers? Could your care-receiver just be tired from not having had enough sleep the night before? First, determine the cause of their anger and then work on a solution. Perhaps taking your loved one to a quieter place or simply breaking down a task that would be easier for them to handle would prove the key to calming them. Think cause and solution whenever confronted with a puzzling outburst.

Anxiety:

Anxiety is generally caused in the average person by difficulty in processing information and experiences. Now, just imagine how unsettling this emotion can be for a person struggling with a damaged brain and, therefore, unable to reason what is happening to them. Much is new and different, while at other times, your loved one is confounded by memories just out of their grasp. This anxiety can cause sleeplessness and restlessness, but it can also cause a seemingly irrational attachment to objects, people, or places.

Strategy:

Reassurance is key to soothing an anxiety-ridden loved one, whether they have dementia or not. Try calming your care-receiver with not only patience and reassurance but distractions. Turning their attention away from their concern to peaceful activities, or things they especially love, will often be enough to calm them. If possible, neutralize their worry with joy, which will result in the benefit of making you feel better as well.

Depression:

Depression affects many people either long-term or occasionally depending upon circumstances during their lifetime. Illness is often one of the driving forces of depression and the illness of dementia is no different. However, the expression of dementia-related depression involves apathy, agitation, insomnia, and delusions, like general depression, but not the loss of self-esteem and suicidal tendencies.

Strategy:

Treating depression in a person suffering from dementia isn't different from trying to cope with the condition of any loved one. It takes patience and compassion and a sincere attempt to help them with a sense of well-being. But when your care-receiver doesn't respond to sincere consideration and gentle prodding, it may be time for medication. Be certain to speak with your loved one's doctor and a mental health specialist you may know so that they will be able to guide you in treating the condition.

Mood Swings:

We all have periodic good and bad days but most of us can reason through why and what to do about it. Those suffering from dementia have the extra added burden of not being able to understand their feelings. Additionally, this is often exacerbated by a fear that comes with the loss of cognitive reasoning; they know something is wrong, but they're not sure why. In a chain of reactions, this can cause anger and lashing out, when the initial problem may be nothing more than general discomfort in their surroundings, lack of sleep, or simply boredom.

Strategy:

To avoid mood swings, learn as much as you can about your care-receiver's triggers; what seems to repeatedly set them off. Learn their likes and dislikes and keep a journal of their reactions until a pattern becomes clear. Things that may not have bothered your loved one in the past, may one day become problematic. Try soothing them with a favorite activity, a song they may especially like, or a nourishing treat. Try to anticipate your care-receiver's reactions; it will help to minimize frustration and embarrassment for both of you.

Strategies for Managing a Patient's Problematic Behavior

The list below is in alphabetical order for ease in finding the particular situation you're addressing. Each patient's progression through the disease is different so there is no order to when, or if, some of these problems may occur.

Aggression:

Even the most mild-mannered of people suffering from dementia can become aggressive when dealing with the frustrations of the disease. Very often, care-receivers lose their ability to communicate their feelings and needs, which can cause them to act out either verbally or physically.

Strategy:

In the moment, first make sure both you and your loved one are safe. Do anything necessary to avoid physical harm and destruction to property and possessions. Then, try to remain calm to elicit composure in your care-receiver. Acknowledge their feelings and provide reassurance that you are there to support them. Most importantly, attempt to figure out what prompted the outburst and try to avoid a repeat in the future.

Hoarding:

Many people experiencing the loss of control that comes with dementia attempt to accumulate things they believe they may need, or which are important to them. They create a private supply of things in places that were comfortable to them earlier in life. This generally isn't a major problem unless food spoilage is involved or the items being hidden do not belong to the care-receiver.

Strategy:

As a harmless behavior, try not to correct or confront your loved one, unless the behavior is destructive, excessive, or at the expense of someone else. Be aware of hiding places and check them regularly. Places like dresser drawers, underneath mattresses, in laundry, and even the trash, are often favorites. Limit access to unnecessary items without making them feel deprived.

Incontinence:

Among the most troubling of all dementia's expressions is the decrease in bladder and bowel control. This usually occurs in the later stages of the disease. This can also happen at any time due to simple difficulties like not remembering where bathroom facilities are or how to use them. Making matters worse, incontinence not only causes inconvenience but embarrassment, which can affect the mood and cooperation of your care-receiver.

Strategy:

Try to make using the restroom as convenient as possible for your loved one. If feasible, move their bed closer to the bathroom at home and sit close to public facilities when able. Schedule regular bathroom breaks and have your care-receiver wear easily removable clothes and diapers.

Profane Language:

The lack of impulse control can often result in your loved one swearing or cursing even if they never did before the onset of the disease. This is often troubling and embarrassing, especially in public.

Strategy:

As unsettling as episodes of swearing can be, keep in mind that this is the disease talking and not the person you love. Remain calm and caring and do what you can to change the situation. Distract your care-receiver by engaging them in a conversation or activity.

Refusing Help:

As with the difficulty in getting your care-receiver to wear diapers, those experiencing dementia may not always be accepting of help. General confusion and mistrust brought on by fear may result in your loved one being resistant to support of any kind or may accept help from only specific individuals, like you. This can leave you, as the only person to which they will respond, especially burdened.

Strategy:

Keeping a set routine is key to your loved one accepting support so that his/her life is made as simple as possible. Learn the ways in which your care-receiver feels comforted and at ease. It may be through simple, gentle touch, a specific phrase, or a method of distraction.

Repetition:

Repeating the same phrase or action can be due to unsettled feelings or simply a lack of forgetting from moment to moment what has been said or done. They may repeat a question because they can't recall having asked it before.

Strategy:

Distraction is the best way to handle these behaviors. Redirect your loved one to another train of thought they seem to enjoy. You can also engage them in some useful or harmless activity until she/he is more emotionally settled.

Sleep Disturbances:

It is not uncommon for people with dementia to have trouble sleeping. As the disease progresses you may find that your loved one sleeps for long periods during the day and is up most of the night. This upside-down behavior may be due to changes in the brain as well as adjustments to a different lifestyle routine.

Strategy:

Attempt to keep to a strict sleep routine every day, including weekends. Use natural light as your guide, waking your loved one with the sunrise and slowly preparing them for bed after dark. Try to avoid naps during the day and excitement too close to bedtime. Avoid all caffeinated food and drink. Simple daily exercise, like a walk in fresh air early in the day, can contribute to better sleep at night. When all else fails, you might want to try CBD supplements, which have been known to improve sleep.

Sundowning:

Some studies reflect that up to 20% of dementia suffers experience increased disorientation and agitation at dusk. This is known as "sundowning," which is not uncommon. They may be due to a problem with your loved one's biological clock or just fatigue from an overly stressful day. Although it is basically harmless, it can be emotionally unsettling to both you and your loved one.

Strategy:

Calming reassurance is one of the best ways to alleviate sundowning. Whether through a soothing touch or supportive phrase, letting your loved one know you care and that you are there for them will help to put them at greater ease. It may also help to close out the dimming light with curtains or blinds, and turn on indoor lighting, as well as distracting your care-receiver with activities they enjoy.

Wandering:

It has been estimated that six out of ten people with dementia wander. This is a staggering number and episodes cannot only cause distress to you but a danger to your loved one. Wandering may be driven by emotional needs like anxiety or boredom, or physical discomforts like hunger and thirst. But, out of confusion, they may also set out looking for someone or falsely believe they are meant to be somewhere else.

Strategy:

As the most potentially serious of all behaviors, it is important that you keep a close eye on your care-receiver. They should not be left unattended. Doors should be kept locked and car keys out of sight. It is worthwhile to invest in tracking devices and identification bracelets and ask neighbors to help keep an eye out for your loved one leaving the house unattended. Most importantly, try to figure out triggers or specific times of the day for their wandering and fill those with activities enjoyable to you both.

Strategies for Managing the Caregiver's Emotional Challenges

Caregivers are slowly losing the people they knew, the relationships they had, and the lives they shared before they needed to provide care.

Caregiving takes more than love. Many skills are required: Communication, collaboration, teamwork, organization, planning, questioning, and more. Very few of us are born with all these skills that take time and effort to acquire.

Potential emotions caregivers encounter:

Anger:

Most times your role is not acknowledged and taken for granted. This is especially painful when you may be caring for an agitated or aggressive person. Simultaneously, you may be dealing with the grief of losing a loved one to a disease. You are not always in a position where you can stop or control these situations making you feel helpless and isolated.

Strategy:

The first thing to realize is that anger is a normal reaction. Caregiver fatigue is the result of daily physical and emotional exhaustion. Forgive yourself, be kind to yourself. It's a sure indication that you need a respite.

Anxiety:

This is one of the most common and pervasive disorders experienced by caregivers. Fear of a loved one's well-being, and their future can be extremely overwhelming for caregivers which results in anxiety and stress.

Strategy:

Chronic worrying is a mental habit you can learn how to break. Practicing relaxation techniques, such as deep breathing, can lower the physical symptoms and mental stress associated with anxiety. Realize that no one can predict the future or control the outcome of every situation. Avoid things that can aggravate the symptoms of anxiety disorders, such as poor diet, caffeine, sugar, smoking, over-the-counter cold medications, and alcohol.

Boredom:

Being trapped in your own home is not healthy. It's natural that you become uninspired and bored. Your world is shrinking, and you have no idea how long this condition will last. Boredom can result in mental, emotional, and physical challenges.

Strategy:

The caregiver needs a break. Whether it's lunch with friends, going for a walk, or just taking a nap. Arrange for a family member, friend, or neighbor to take your place for a few hours or an afternoon. People like to help, especially if they know it's for only a short time and not every day. Give them an opportunity to do a charitable kindness.

Depression:

Caregivers are always at risk for depression. Feeling helpless, hopeless, and alone over a long period of time can all contribute to the possibility of becoming depressed. If you find yourself tearful, sleepless, and unable to enjoy your normal activities then you may have a depression.

Strategy:

Depression is treatable. It is helpful to eat properly and exercise to reduce your depression. If this strategy does not help, ask your family physician or a mental health care provider for assistance. Some counselors and support groups specialize in caregiver issues and are a great resource.

Disgust:

Daily toileting is an extraordinary event for most amateur caregivers. As dementia disease progresses, incontinence increases, and adult diaper changes can be nauseating and repulsive. Changing a parent, grandparent, or father-in-law can be unnerving and uncomfortable. Drooling, sloppy eating, and poor personal care can also cause feelings of disgust.

Strategy:

First, we must accept that the care-receiver is not in control of these behaviors. We also must acknowledge that toileting and bathing will always be an important part of this kind of caregiving. Support groups will help with some good tips because they all have the same issue. It may help to contact a hospice in your area because they have some of the best trained professionals.

Finding ways to minimize your need to do personal care tasks including incontinence care is vital to weathering your caregiver journey, which could stretch on for years. If possible, hire an attendant to do routine care or have someone from the family do these things who might cope better.

Embarrassment:

Dementia patients may make a scene or make impolite comments in public places. Sometimes they may scream in restaurants or have bad odors. Most family members and caregivers feel responsible and make excuses or just leave.

Strategy:

When in a restaurant it is best to alert the server or management that you have an impaired guest that might make a scene and you will do your best to control them. You will find that they will usually take the initiative to alert surrounding tables and most likely they will be supportive. Some caregivers create small business cards which read, "My loved one has dementia and can no longer control their behavior" to be distributed to those around them when appropriate.

Fear:

There are many reasons fear occurs in caregiving. There are also many side-effects of fear that include feelings of anger, resentment, and bitterness that increases caregiver stress. Fear piled on top of negative feelings reduces motivation to act. Caregivers who experience fear and denial are quick to eliminate options and close their minds to actions that have been proven to work. Fear of the "what-ifs" can paralyze caregivers.

Strategy:

Having a backup caregiver in place in case something happens to you can be very comforting. Make a list of all medications and procedures to be followed if an emergency happens while you are gone. It pays to develop an ongoing network of family and friends who will be there when you most need them. An extended support group doesn't require an orientation each time there is an event. Most people like to be helpful and part of a team. Don't isolate yourself. Invite your whole team to your home for coffee and discussions about the progress of your loved one. This connection will eliminate the confusion when an emergency arises.

Frustration:

It's normal to get frustrated after months or years of a constant routine when dealing with a sick loved one who is usually deteriorating instead of getting well. Sometimes it feels as if you can't do anything right. This can lead to losing your temper, overeating, and substance abuse.

Strategy:

Be aware that it is going to happen so acknowledge it. Then focus on your own health. Become proactive with a diet program and exercise routine. Join a dementia support group where you can vent your frustration with people who are experiencing the same feelings.

Grief:

It is heartbreaking to watch your loved one slowly decline and know there is no cure. You are only capable of being there for them, keeping them comfortable, clean, and hopefully free of pain. Grieving is a natural process in this situation, and it should be acknowledged daily.

Strategy:

There is a tendency to avoid the sadness that comes with grief, but allowing ourselves to feel the grief promotes healing. It's best to confront it. Some caregivers make a list of all the things their loved one enjoyed and cross them off as the disease progresses.

Impatience:

As dementia progresses, you may find your loved one resisting normal routines. Everything slows down, from getting out of bed, to dressing, eating, leaving for doctor appointments, etc. This constant treadmill can lead to frustration and anger that turns bitter like a virus that spreads within the caregiver causing further emotional and physical damage. This can lead to caregiver "burnout." Caregivers become overwhelmed and are physically, emotionally, and mentally exhausted from the stress and burden of caring for their loved one. Some of the physical signs to recognize are fatigue, frequent headaches, increase or decrease in appetite, unusual change in weight, and insomnia. Emotional signs to recognize are feeling anxious, becoming angry and argumentative, being easily irritated, constant worrying, hopelessness, impatience, feeling depressed, not able to concentrate, and lacking motivation.

Strategy:

If available, consider respite care. Using respite care for a few hours to a few weeks is an option in many places. When you need a few hours or a day for yourself, in-home services, such as a home health aide or an adult day center, can take care of your loved one. The drawback is that you pay a fee for these services that usually isn't covered by Medicare or insurance. Be honest with yourself. Know what you can and cannot do, and delegate the rest to others.

Ask for help from family and friends or a support group. Pay attention to your feelings and needs, take regular breaks, try to maintain social activities, exercise, and have a planned sleep schedule.

Jealousy:

Jealousy is a complicated human emotion. In many ways, it is based on love, hate, paranoia, insecurity, self-hate, and low self-esteem.

Jealousy is no stranger to caregiving. The caregiver could be jealous of others who can socialize and enjoy life while they cares for their homebound spouse, who has late-stage dementia. Some caregivers must leave jobs to undertake caregiving duties and are envious of colleagues able to pursue their career dreams. Those without family support are envious of those with it.

Many spouses become jealous of hired caregivers. A younger, more attractive woman caring for a husband may be accused of trying to steal him.

Strategy:

Find new self-appreciation. The best antidote to a caregiver envy is greater self-regard. Lots of caregivers who have mastered caregiving's many challenges find that making a significant difference for someone they love has led to increased gratification and a greater sense of purpose. They may still compare themselves to others but perhaps only to note that non-caregivers haven't yet had the opportunity to step up, muster their strengths, and prove their mettle.

Recognize your jealousy. When we name the jealousy, it loses its power, because we are no longer letting it shame us. Tell yourself that you don't need this emotion in your life, and you're relinquishing it. Many times, jealously raises its ugly head when we are tired or sick ourselves while caring for another.

Loneliness:

Caregiver isolation and loneliness have serious implications on our mental and physical health.

Loneliness and social isolation can take a steep toll on the human body. Studies show that people who are chronically lonely have more heart disease, and are more vulnerable to metastatic cancer and strokes. They may also be more likely to develop neurodegenerative diseases such as Alzheimer's.

Lonely adults are 25% more likely to die prematurely. Elderly people who are lonely die at twice the rate as those who are socially connected.

Caregiving for a dementia patient is a 24/7 task that usually results in living in a world of silence. For many of us, conversation, which was a routine part of our daily lives, may slowly diminish while caring for a dementia patient. Since many senior caregivers are not computer users, they would not have the option of going online to relate to family or friends.

Strategy:

Meditation: Even if one does not have time to get to a church or synagogue service, spending time in prayer or meditation or even listening to calming music can have a beneficial effect on one's body, mind, and spirit and can leave one feeling renewed and re-energized.

Caregivers Support Group: Meeting with people who are having a similar experience and can share ideas on how to deal with loneliness is important.

Online Support Group Network: This is a great option when there are no in-person groups in your area. AARP offers guidance and support on their Family Caregiving site as well as on their Care Connection.

Dementia Day Care Centers: If available in your area, they can usually care for your loved one for up to eight hours a day. This can allow time to reconnect with family and friends. Enlist the help of friends and family. When people offer to help, stop refusing! Some people are embarrassed to admit that they might need help, afraid to appear "needy", or think it is too much trouble to let people help.

The Reluctant Caregiver

According to the Department of Health and Human Services, there are 44 million people caring for loved ones in the United States. How do these millions of caregivers survive the emotional, physical, and financial burdens of caregiving? Do they freely choose this burden?

Family caregiving is usually an unwelcome challenge that is thrust upon the closest family member depending on their ability, location, or availability. Accepting the task means a complete change to that person's lifestyle and future plans. Caring for an Alzheimer's or dementia patient is one of the most demanding types of care. The patient has no chance of recovery, the challenges increase with each new stage of the disease, and the end is predictable. Caring for someone from five to fifteen years is not uncommon.

Few family caregivers have training or knowledge of what will be demanded of them. This may lead to guilt, mistakes, and possible judgement from other family members. Also, some past family interactions may not have been pleasant. Many times, it intensifies the feelings and drudges up painful memories that impacts the quality of care.

Understand, that if it is an elderly caregiver, they are aging with the patient and are susceptible to many of the normal aging maladies. Therefore, it's reasonable to conclude that the quality of care would also diminish with the passage of time. Also, the constant fear—*if I die, who will take care of my spouse or parent?* is always present.

Many caregivers present an outward resilience to hide their inner feelings, so it is difficult to evaluate how they are coping.

To determine how reluctant caregivers feel about their new calling, we resorted to surveying a number of anonymous readers' comments in the book review section of caregiver books.

Below, in their own words are reviews which are unedited for spelling and grammar:
"Sadly, caregiver-shaming has forced some of us to go underground. There are secret groups on Facebook where caregivers meet during the insomniac hours to share and vent what we feel freely. We even have "Throat Punch Thursdays" — where we rage on the doctors who don't call us back, the pharmacies that can't figure out how to submit a bill to insurance, the morass that is Medicare and Medicaid and VA benefits that no one

understands. And yes, sometimes we throat punch our patients. "I just wanted to go to the supermarket alone and walk up and down every aisle — alone. But he wanted to come along. Dammit." Sometimes, we could use a little care ourselves and we find it best among strangers who don't shame us for being open with our feelings.

In the judgment-free zone of Facebook — bet you didn't know such a thing existed — we get to say things like: "We don't feel honored. We don't feel lucky. We can't even love the same." Roll those words around your tongue like a fine wine and then let me know how you think we should feel."

"When I complain about taking care of my mother-in-law, know that it is in the context of having a broken spirit. It comes from having everything go wrong in the past 13 years. It comes from being tired of losing everything and everyone. I am in a place where all I want is to live a nice quiet life with my husband without any major changes. I don't want to be taking care of anyone but myself."

"If you could stop judging us for a minute, you might realize that every honest caregiver has moments of sheer rage and resentment. One woman I know goes down to her basement and screams into a pillow, so her kids don't hear. Me? I prefer the shower, the one in the bathroom where the door still locks. Why can't a caregiver just say, "I really can't take this much more" without someone telling her she is wrong?"

"Caregivers feel sad, lost, and sometimes angry — very angry. Since I began writing about my caregiving experience. I have heard from caregivers who say they sometimes wish their patient were dead. "Then I could just have a normal life," said one woman who's been caregiving for almost three years without a day off."

"I just can't catch a break. When is it my turn to live again?"

A caregiver friend — half my age and with twice my smarts — says that what she longs for most is a single day in which all the decisions don't fall to her. "It would be a mini-vacation," she said. She would also like people to stop telling her what a great job she's doing. "Good job" Good job!" she mimics. "It's like I'm in second grade and just got all my spelling words right." There are days when I wish my husband would just try harder. Sometimes it's like I'm the only one vested in his care. Why can't he take the meds like the doctor tells him to? Why is every doctor 'an idiot'?"

"Yep — sometimes our patients don't put their own oars in the water, and we are out there paddling alone — paddling alone for them. Invariably, we think, "If he doesn't care, why should I?" The front door is all that stands between us and freedom and don't think we don't eye it."

"Also, please don't suggest that we need therapy to learn how to cope better. We aren't what's wrong and in need of fixing. What's wrong is that even though family caregivers save the country $500 billion a year by providing our services for free, nobody is out there trying to make our lives a little easier. But instead of solid counsel, all we get is your view of how you think we should be feeling."

"It takes a special heart to be a caregiver in general. It takes an incredible inward surrender to God and the leadership and guidance of His Spirit to be a caregiver to someone who has wronged you in pretty major ways. The author offers a unique perspective and serves an example for navigating through such tough circumstances."

"I do have an aide from hospice coming in 2X a week to bathe mother in her bed. The nurse comes once a week just to check vitals and see if I have any questions about mother's condition. I have been looking into a day provider who can come in 4 – 6 hours a week to sit with Mom so I can go out and spend some "me" time, but the cost is kind of high — $18.50 an hour. They charge a flat fee whether the aide does any housework or not on top of watching Mom. I am looking into other companies now who can provide the same service at a cheaper rate. That $18.50/hr. is steep.

To help with my emotional well-being I have been spending my mornings in Bible study (which by the tone of my last post was needed for sure!) and I have been working on my attitude. It is one thing to do what I believe is the will of God out of obligation and entirely another to do what I think is God's will with a wiling heart. I can look back and see over the last 3 – 4 months I was operating in a spirit of obligation and not grace. Thankfully, God has made my mother's disposition so cute it is difficult to remain angry at the situation. There are many times a day she says or does something that is kind of adorable and it does help me to enjoy caring for her. I am even doing waaaay better with the bowel incontinence which is truly a never-ending battle, but for now, I am managing it instead of allowing it to manage me.

She is still in hospice, but it doesn't seem like she's going to pass away anytime soon so it's kind of a perplexing situation. There is some declining every 2 – 3 months but not the all-out decline I was expecting when she waited into the hospice program. I really didn't think my mother would still be here. I thought she would pass in October/November but she is still with us. It's both troubling and surprising. I mean, could she really live another 6 – 8 years like this? Dear gawd. I hope not. Not like this, God please, not like this. The lack of mobility and diaper changes and having to feed her is such a responsibility and it stealing from my duties as a wife. Time will tell though won't it?"

"This book was recommended by my brother's doctor for me to read to help me find a better way to interact with him while he is living with Dementia with Lewy Bodies. Maybe it's because I've been dealing with this for more than 3 years with him, or maybe it's just the differences between Alzheimer's disease and DLB, but I found most of the book to be condescending and blaming of the "care partners"."

"One passage that really stands out deals with how to deal with aggressive behavior. In the example, the caregiver walked up behind a patient and put a bowl of soup on the table. The patient then reacts badly, throws the bowl of soup at the caregiver, along with a magazine. The author goes on to explain that the patient's behavior was *obviously* the fault of the caregiver (a recurring theme throughout the book) and if the caregiver had just behaved differently, the patient wouldn't have acted aggressively.

Another example of bizarre advice is about a patient who tries to open the car door while the car is going down the road. The solution? Don't take the patient anywhere in the car. Now...this begs the question...how you get the patient to Doctor appointments, daycare, etc. if you can't drive them? Even if bus service were available everywhere, putting a person with dementia onto a bus full of people is a terrifying thought."

Caregiver Burnout

Caregivers have feelings of helplessness, stress, anger, and depression. Sometimes they feel imprisoned by their informal job of caring for an elderly family member. They often develop increased health problems related to these feeling. Many times, it leads to depression. Depression is a real illness and carries with it a high cost in terms of relationship problems, family suffering, and lost work productivity.

Depression is more than just sadness. People with depression may experience a lack of interest and pleasure in daily activities, and significant weight loss or gain. It is a highly treatable illness, with psychotherapy, cognitive-behavioral techniques, and medication.

SECTION TWO

CHAPTER 3

Caring Guidelines

Breaking the News

When it's time to tell the diagnosed patient, consider doing so with the help of a physician or other professional. Make sure there is ample time for questions and coming to terms with the diagnosis. It's also best to give your loved one time to digest the news before you break it to other family and friends. Encourage family members and friends to participate in the loved one's care.

If you are responsible for caring for a loved one who has just been diagnosed with Alzheimer's, you are probably also responsible for sharing the diagnosis with other family members. It's not easy news to share, and with it comes the realization that life is unlikely to ever be the same.

Taking the Car Keys

Discussing a loved one's need to stop driving is one of the most difficult discussions you may ever face. Seniors are reluctant to give up driving because it is one of the few ways they can continue to feel independent. The discussion becomes even more difficult when the person still maintains most of his or her faculties, just not those that enable safe driving.

The following few ideas might help your discussion.

- Be empathetic—don't confront them with all the negatives.
- Keep the conversation non-accusatory, honest, and between "adults," not "child and parent." Say things like, "We are concerned," "We care," or "We don't want you to get hurt or to hurt others."
- Don't approach this subject as though a conclusion has already been made.
- If you can, avoid an immediate cutoff time. Do what you can to limit driving in small ways over time.
- Help the senior make a schedule. He or she can plan activities and arrange alternative means of transportation.

Elder Mistreatment

Dementia and Elder Mistreatment

National Center for Elder Abuse

Older people with dementia are particularly susceptible to abuse. Nearly one in two older adults with cognitive impairment experiences abuse. In addition to being dependent upon others for assistance, elders with dementia are more likely to experience deficits in memory, communication, and judgment that make it harder for them to identify, prevent, and report mistreatment. Many may also be reluctant to report abuse by caregivers and others upon whom they rely. Older people with dementia are often at an increased risk of mistreatment because of pre-existing medical and mental health weaknesses.

The most frequently observed signs of mistreatment are referenced below. Please note that indications of abuse may present differently based upon multiple factors, including the type, degree, duration, and context of abuse experienced. Manifestations of abuse may also be impacted by the older adult's physical and cognitive condition, social connectedness, and emotional state.

<u>Psychological Abuse</u>

- Emotional distress or agitation
- Withdrawal from activities of daily life
- Uncommunicative or non-responsive
- Unusual behaviors commonly attributed to dementia (e.g. sucking, biting, rocking)
- Lack of self-care
- Lower self-esteem, feelings of despair, or a sense of worthlessness

<u>Physical Abuse</u>

- Bruises, abrasions, welts, lacerations, or rope marks
- Head trauma or bone fractures

- Open wounds, cuts, punctures, or untreated injuries in various stages of healing
- Sprains, dislocations, and internal injuries/bleeding
- Bite, strangulation, burn marks, or patterns of injury
- Falls, including broken eyeglasses or frames
- Physical indications of punishment, including evidence of physical restraints
- Medication overdose or chemical restraints
- Sudden behavioral changes

Financial Abuse

- Sudden changes in bank account or banking practices, including an unexplained withdrawal of large sums of money or the addition of signatories to an older person's bank signature card
- Abrupt changes to a will or other financial documents
- The unexplained disappearance of funds or valuable possessions, or sudden transfer of assets
- Substandard care provision, unpaid bills, or eviction proceedings
- The provision of unnecessary services
- Depression or anxiety
- Evidence of poor financial decision-making
- Malnutrition

Neglect

- Dehydration or malnutrition
- Untreated bed sores
- Poor personal hygiene
- Unattended or untreated health problems
- Unsafe living conditions
- Unsanitary living conditions

Sexual Abuse

- Bruises, abrasions, or lacerations around the breasts or genital area
- Unexplained sexually transmitted disease or genital infection
- Unexplained vaginal or anal bleeding or incontinence
- Increased anxiety or depressive symptoms
- Sleep disturbances, agitation, or restlessness

Abuse in Institutional Settings

Older residents of long-term care facilities who have disabilities or otherwise experience frailties may be at heightened risk of mistreatment and less able to safeguard themselves from environmental harm or extricate themselves from danger. Abuse within institutions may be observed in the forms outlined above but may also be discerned in other ways. For example, physical abuse may appear as hygiene neglect, which results in skin abrasions and breakdown, such as pressure ulcers. Other means of institutional abuse are medication withholding, food deprivation, treatment neglect, and chemical restraints. Psychological mistreatment may be also employed and expressed as threats of death or harm.

Dehydration

Dehydration occurs when more water is moving out of the cells in our bodies then what we are taking in. Our bodies are over 50% water, and we need it for blood to flow and for our organs to function. When we lose too much water from not drinking enough, sweating, or illness, we can get dehydrated. In the elderly this is quite common.

Dehydration affects people of all ages, but adults aged sixty-five years and over have a greater risk. About 40% of seniors are not hydrated enough and therefore are at more risk. These challenges are more likely because many elders have other underlying health problems.

Some elder problems:

- Memory problems like dementia can cause elders to forget to drink.
- Lack of mobility can prevent seniors from getting water.

- Difficulty with swallowing and bladder and bowel control (incontinence) contributes to dehydration.
- Medications can also cause dehydration. The interactions of multiple medications are a serious issue that should be discussed with a doctor.
- Declining kidney function can cause problems.
- Decreased thirst is a factor. The ability to detect and respond to thirst decreases with age.

Signs that an elder may be experiencing dehydration include:

- Fatigue
- Headaches
- Dry mouth/cracked lips
- Dizziness
- Confusion
- Muscle cramping in arms and legs
- Nausea
- Agitation
- Changes in urination frequency or strong-smelling urine.

Dehydration Prevention:

- Don't assume that someone with dementia will ask for a drink.
- Keep small glasses of water on tables around the house — near the chair, the bedside table, the bathroom sinks, and the kitchen table.
- Ice cream snacks
- Broth-based soups
- Jell-O
- Sports drinks
- Thickener can be added to water and other liquids to reduce the risk of choking.

Addressing Pain

Pain is now considered the fifth vital sign, yet it is often overlooked in the person with dementia. Caregivers or family members may not be certain if the person is in pain, thus delaying appropriate intervention strategies. Often, dementia-related behaviors emerge due to the lack of assessment and treatment of painful conditions. While self-reporting is always considered first, people in the advanced or terminal stage of dementia may need to be assessed using pain behavioral assessment tools.

Each person with dementia deserves a pain evaluation and subsequent treatment and all care needs to be individualized. If there is any indication that a person has pain, it is important to assume pain is present.

Hiring a nursing assistant (CNA)

Certified Nursing Assistants (CNA) are responsible for many patient-care tasks to ensure that each patient receives the comprehensive and personalized care they need.

They often have the following responsibilities:

- Grooming and bathing patients with low mobility
- Preparing each patient room with necessary items like blankets, pillows, medical equipment, and bathroom needs
- Helping patients eat and take medications
- Making sure they have regular meals and proper medication dosages
- Monitoring vitals and patient behavior and reporting them to the nursing and medical staff
- Assisting patients with mobility needs; transferring them from wheelchair to bed
- Turning or adjusting patients in bed to prevent bedsores or other discomfort
- Exercising patients by helping them walk

Medications

Why monitoring is necessary

When someone with dementia begins making medication mistakes, it's a sign for the caregiver to start monitoring prescription intake. Forgetting to take daily medications can be detrimental to the person's overall health, especially if doses are missed on a frequent basis. Someone with Alzheimer's might also forget having already taken a scheduled dosage and accidentally take it again, potentially more than once, leading to life-threatening overdoses. Additionally, seniors may inadvertently take incorrect medications—a family member's prescription, perhaps—which could expose them to dangerous side effects.

Many people—even those without memory problems—find that common pill organizers are helpful. Most dispensers include day-of-the-week compartments, and some have morning and nighttime separators. There are even automated dispensers that track activity and send reminders via text messages.

Also, always be certain to properly store meds between doses. Never leave drugs on countertops or in cabinets where someone with dementia might find and take them.

If you notice sudden changes in the health of the person in your charge (i.e., bathroom accidents, behavioral outbursts), notify a doctor immediately. Such changes could indicate an adverse reaction to a medication or be symptoms of a new illness.

The National Institute on aging recommends the following to stay on track with medicines:

- Keep a list of all medicines in a safe place.
- Bring the list when you talk to the doctor or pharmacist.
- Use a pillbox.
- Put notes around the house to remind them to take their medicines each day.
- Talk to their doctor about all the medicines, remedies, and vitamins they use. Include any medicines without a prescription. These are called OTC (over the counter) medicines. OTC drugs include things like cough syrup for a cold and antacid for an upset stomach.

Write down:

- the drug name, the doctor who prescribed it, and how much to take
- the name and amount of each remedy, vitamin, and OTC drug taken
- the time of day to take each medicine

Talk to your doctor about any side effects before stopping any medicines. The doctor may have tips that can help, such as eating a light snack with pills. You may want to talk to the doctor about switching the patient to a new medicine.

Ask your doctor:

- What is the name of the medicine and why are they taking it?
- What medical condition does this medicine treat?
- How many times a day should the patient take this medicine? What is the dosage?
- How long will it take this medicine to work?
- What should I do if they miss a dose?
- Are there any side effects I should know about? When should I call you if the patient is having side effects?
- Can I safely mix this medicine with the remedies, vitamins, and OTC drugs?

Before you leave the pharmacy, be sure to:

- Make sure the label has the correct name on it.
- Make sure you can read and understand the directions on the bottle.
- Make sure the directions are the same as your doctor's. If not, tell the pharmacist.
- Ask for an easy-open cap if you have trouble opening the bottle. Be sure to keep all medicines out of reach of children.
- Find out if the medicine needs be stored in a special place, such as the refrigerator.
- Should the medicine be taken with food? Are there any liquids or foods which should be avoided with this medication?
- Is there a generic (non-brand name) version of the drug?

Dentistry

Good dental hygiene is one of the daily habits that is often neglected by those who are cognitively impaired. Poor oral hygiene, difficulty wearing dentures, and the inability to carry out normal oral hygiene procedures usually cause impaired oral health in people with Alzheimer's disease. There are some common issues people with Alzheimer's may experience. These patients may not remember to brush their teeth or forget how to use a toothbrush and toothpaste. It can also be more difficult to notice if someone with Alzheimer's is experiencing mouth pain.

Some common dental issues to look for at dental check-ups include:

- If a dental care routine is neglected, bacteria can begin to build up and wear away the enamel causing cavities. If ignored, broken teeth can cause more serious infections in the mouth.
- An abscessed tooth is an infection inside the tooth that can spread to the gums. It's very painful and can spread quickly causing an abscess.
- Dry mouth is a common symptom seen in patients with Alzheimer's caused by the mouth not making enough saliva and can lead to ulcers, sores, and cavities.
- Bad breath can be caused by poor dental hygiene, dry mouth, infections, medications, and certain foods.
- Gum disease results in tooth loss, which often leads to problems with chewing, swallowing, and food selection. It's difficult to absorb nutrients from food efficiently if it is not chewed well.

Periodontal disease is also associated with weight loss and wasting, which might contribute to cognitive decline. Evidence from several studies indicates deterioration in nutritional status in individuals missing teeth.

Because of these issues, it's important for somebody with Alzheimer's to try and maintain a daily oral care routine as well as receive regular cleanings and exams from a dental professional.

We typically brush our teeth in the bathroom. However, if it's more comfortable for someone to brush while sitting down on a chair, simply provide a plastic tub and glass of water for the patient. Some caregivers encourage the patient to "watch me" and sit across from their loved one with their own tub and toothbrush and start brushing their own teeth. Many times, this will stimulate their partner to follow.

Don't use fluoride toothpaste if the patient is inclined to swallow it. If the patient doesn't like toothpaste, try using baking soda and water, or just plain water.

If you can trust the patient not to swallow mouthwash, try an anti-plaque mouthwash when brushing is not feasible.

Ask your dentist about using a super soft toothbrush or one with a sponge head instead of a bristle head.

Provide a toothbrush with a large handle.

Flossing is almost impossible. Buy a "GUM Proxabush Go-Betweens." As they are clinically designed to go between teeth and are a safe, easy way to clean teeth, bridges and dental implants.

Clearly and gently tell them what you want to do. Try to touch their mouth with the toothbrush and see if they'll let you slip it in. Don't force the toothbrush in. Sometimes, just asking them to smile will make them open their mouth. If they open wide, brush the back teeth first, since these are the hardest to clean.

Some days, it may be too difficult and that's okay. If this happens, try again tomorrow. Experiment with different methods to find what works best.

Care of Dentures

If your loved one wears dentures, you should take them out of their mouth for at least four to eight hours every day. Clean them and then store them in a cup or bowl filled with water. Never use toothpaste on dentures, as this can damage them. Instead, rinse them under running water and brush with a wet toothbrush.

On your first dentist visit:

- Bring the insurance card (if applicable)
- Bring the patient's identification card
- Bring a list of medication that they are currently taking
- On the first visit expect to have a full mouth set of X-rays taken. If the patient has had a full mouth X-ray taken in the last year, please have the previous dentist forward them in advance by mail or email.

SECTION 3

CHAPTER 4

Responsible Planning

Financial and Legal Issues

Plan for care while your loved one is still mentally aware enough to make decisions. What end of life medical treatments does your loved one desire or not want when they're no longer able to speak for themselves? Designate someone to be a healthcare proxy who will make healthcare decisions when the care-receiver is unable to communicate.

The plan should include the following:

- A will
- A living will declaration
- A living trust, either revocable or irrevocable
- A medical directive
- A health care power of attorney
- A durable power of attorney
- A do-not-resuscitate (DNR) order

The person with the durable power of attorney will need personal information in order to perform their duties. They should have access to the following:

- Computer login & passwords
- Insurance policies
- Investment statements
- Any bond or stock certificate
- Property deeds, mortgages, etc.

- Bank loan documents
- Credit cards
- Memberships
- Newspaper and magazine subscriptions
- Name of attorney and accountant

Alzheimer's and related Dementias Education and Referral (ADEAR) Center
800-438-4380
adear@nia.nih.gov
www.nia.nih.gov/alzheimers

alzheimers.gov
www.alzheimers.gov
AARP 888-687-2277 (toll free)
www.aarpo.org/home-family/caregiving/

Medicare and Medicaid Assistance

Medicaid is health insurance for low-income Americans of all ages. Medicare is health insurance for all Americans, ages sixty-five and older, regardless of their income. Medicaid may cover many long-term non-medical services and supports people with Alzheimer's or other dementias. Although each state offers different long-term care benefits, we will only address general coverage such as personal care or assistance involving bathing, grooming, mobility, toiletry, eating, and transportation. Some states offer assistance with medication management, shopping for essentials, light house-cleaning, and preparing food. Another benefit that may be available is the cost of home modifications, such as widening doorways to allow wheelchair access, installing walk-in showers, and grab bars. Medicaid may also pay for assistive technology, like electronic pill boxes for medication control, or in-home respite care to give caregivers time off from their caregiving duties.

Respite care is provided in the recipient's home on a short-term basis because of the absence or need for relief of the primary caregiver. Medicaid recipients can access in-home support services either through their state's regular Medicaid program or through Home and Community-Based Services (HCBS) Medical Waiver.

Nursing Homes:

Medicaid will cover nursing home care for persons with Alzheimer's or other dementias in all fifty states and Washington D.C. This Medicaid coverage is an entitlement. Medicaid will pay for the room, meals, and care. Not all nursing homes accept Medicaid patients. There are private, pay-only nursing homes. Many nursing homes only accept a limited number of Medicaid beneficiaries.

Center for Medicare and Medicaid Services (CMS)

Home health provisions:

Effective January 2018, CMS implemented the final rule for home health agencies, publishing the new rules those agencies need to meet to be reimbursed by Medicare and Medicaid.

The new rule includes provisions for identifying, engaging, and training family caregivers of home health beneficiaries. It requires home health agencies to identify the family caregiver of the person receiving home health services and include the caregiver's contact information in the person's clinical record. It also requires home health agencies to inform the older person or adult with disabilities of his or her rights, and to notify the individual, family caregiver, and physician if a change to the care plan occurs. The rule requires agencies to evaluate the family caregiver's willingness, ability, availability, and schedule to provide assistance when developing the person's care plan and offers education and training to the family caregiver.

Medicare Part A&B

Home health services

How often is it covered?

Medicare Part A (Hospital Insurance) and/or Medicare Part B (Medical Insurance) cover eligible home health services like these:

- Part-time or "intermittent" skilled nursing care
- Physical therapy
- Occupational therapy
- Speech-language pathology services
- Medical social services
- Part-time or intermittent home health aide services (personal hands-on care)
- Injectable osteoporosis drugs for women

Usually, a home health care agency coordinates the services your doctor orders for you.

Medicare doesn't pay for:
- 24-hour-a-day care at home
- Meals delivered to your home
- Homemaker services (like shopping, cleaning, and laundry) when this is the only care you need
- Custodial or personal care (like bathing, dressing, or using the bathroom) when this is the only care you need

Medicare Hospice Benefit

If someone is eligible for Medicare and is in hospice, their caregivers are eligible for respite under the Medicare Hospice benefit.

State Family Caregiver Support Programs: If your state has a state-funded family caregiver support program, respite funding may be available through this source. Visit the Family Caregiver Alliance Family Care Navigator for more information.

Veterans: Veterans eligible for outpatient medical services can also receive non-institutional respite, outpatient geriatric evaluation and management services and therapeutically oriented outpatient day care. Respite care may be provided in a home or other non-institutional setting, such as a community nursing home. Ordinarily respite is limited to no more than thirty days per year. The services can be contracted or provided directly by the staff of the Veterans Health Administration (VHA) or by another provider or payer. A new program administered by the Department of Veterans Affairs, the Family Caregiver Program established by the Caregivers and Veterans Omnibus Health Services Act of 2010, provides additional support to eligible post-9/11 Veterans who elect to receive their care in a home setting from a primary Family Caregiver. For more information, visit the VA Caregiver Support Program or call the VA Caregiver Support Line at 1-855-260-3274.

Military Families: Military families should look to TRICARE's Extended Care Health Option (ECHO) or the Military Exceptional Family Member Program (EFMP), which offers respite care to anyone in the military who is enrolled in the EFMP and meets the criteria.

Advance Care Planning: Medical Issues to Consider

By Cheryl Arenella, MD, MPH
American Hospice Foundation
(www.americanhospice.org).

What are the varied medical issues that a person should keep in mind in order to be thoughtful and thorough when doing advance care planning? This article will explore several medical options, considering when an intervention is likely to be helpful, when it is unlikely to be helpful, and what the burdens and side effects of a particular intervention are likely to be.

Before getting into an exploration of the medical issues, however, we need to be clear about what is meant by advance care planning.

What is advance care planning?

Advance care planning is a process by which an individual plans for a time in the future when he/she might be unable to make decisions. The person tries to set up a system where his/her treatment preferences will be followed, even if the person is unable to make his/her wishes known at the time.

There are several different types of advance care planning, including:

- A Living Will: A simple statement asking for no heroic care in the case that the person is terminally ill.
- A Values History: A statement of values regarding health care in the event of a life-threatening illness.
- A Medical Directive: A set of instructions based on likely scenarios of illness, goals of care, and specific treatments, usually combined with a general values statement.
- A proxy designation, known as a *Durable Power of Attorney for Health Care* or a *Health Care Proxy*: A formal legal statement naming the person whom the patient wants to make pertinent health care decisions if the patient is unable to do so. A proxy designation often accompanies one or the other of the preceding three instructional directives. The responsibility of the proxy is to make the treatment decisions that the patient would make if he/she were able to express a preference. For this reason, it is imperative that when a person chooses a proxy for health care decisions, the person discusses with the proxy what that person's wishes would be concerning options for treatment interventions.

In order to execute a written instructional advance directive, or to have an informed discussion with the chosen health care proxy, the person doing the advance care planning needs to understand the medical issues that form the basis for making health care decisions.

Some questions to consider when doing advance care planning include:

- Is my medical condition at the time reversible or irreversible?
- Do I at that time have a non-curable chronic medical condition that will progress to end stage disease*?
- Am I in a coma, or a persistent vegetative state?
- Is meaningful recovery possible or unlikely?

*A chronic condition is considered to be "end stage" when optimal medical care can no longer stabilize the medical condition of the person who suffers with the disease. The person has frequent medical decompensations (episodes when the disease worsens to the point that the person requires hospitalization). The disease impacts the person's ability to function in everyday life, and functioning deteriorates over time. The burden of uncomfortable or even painful symptoms on the person is quite high.

Desired interventions will likely differ depending on the answers to the above questions.

In addition, the benefits and the burdens of the intervention will need to be considered:

Help me to live longer?

Improve my quality of life?

Enable me to do more things?

Lessen my suffering?

What kind of burdens and side effects will the proposed treatment impose?

These basic questions can be used in discussions with health care providers to try to clarify various scenarios that may occur in the future.

About the author: Dr. Cheryl Arenella does health care consulting for programs focused on improving end-of-life care. She has over 20 years of experience in the field of Hospice and Palliative Medicine. She is a former trustee of the American Board of Hospice and Palliative Medicine.

COPYRIGHT INFORMATION

The materials on this website are released under the Creative Commons Zero Waiver 1.0 (CC0). You may reproduce all or part of these materials if you cite American Hospice Foundation and link to this website (www.americanhospice.org).

Artificial Nutrition and Hydration at the End of Life: Beneficial or Harmful?

By Cheryl Arenella, MD MPH

This information is provided by American Hospice Foundation (www.americanhospice.org).

Excerpts:

There are few treatment decisions more difficult for families and loved ones to make than those surrounding the use of artificial nutrition and hydration in the seriously or terminally ill person.

But first, let us dispel the myth that artificial nutrition and hydration is not really a medical treatment at all but rather basic care, like giving a meal to someone.

Like many medical interventions, all forms of artificial nutrition and hydration:
- Require the patient to undergo uncomfortable, and at times painful,
- procedures for the treatment to be started;
- Have known side effects and potential complications, including serious infections, fluid overload, nausea/vomiting and diarrhea, electrolyte and mineral imbalances, and even death;
- Have indications (use of the treatment for patients with similar conditions has been usually more beneficial than harmful);
- Have contraindications (use of the treatment for patients with similar conditions has been usually more harmful than beneficial);
- Hold very little similarity to a person sitting with family and socializing while enjoying a tasty meal.

What is meant by "artificial nutrition and hydration"?

Artificial nutrition and/or hydration is a treatment intervention that delivers fluids and/or nutrition by means other than a person taking something in his/her mouth and swallowing it.

Recently the scientific community has taken a closer look at the use of artificial nutrition and hydration to see if there is good evidence that these treatments are useful. There have been some surprising findings! Myths that have been held about the usefulness of artificial nutrition and hydration are being challenged, particularly as they have been used for persons who have incurable disease, in persons who have neurologic or brain disorders, and in the frail elderly person.

What is known about the side effects and complications of artificial nutrition and hydration?

Complications and side effects vary by the type of artificial nutrition and hydration used:

- TPN and central catheters can cause infection at the site of the catheter and in the catheter itself as well as sepsis (a generalized life-threatening infection). Pneumothorax (collapse of the lung) can occur at the time of inserting the catheter. Thrombosis (clots in the vein) can occur, causing local swelling. Sometimes these clots can travel to other parts of the body such as the brain or lung and can be life-threatening. Cardiac arrhythmias (irregularities of the heart beat) as well as electrolyte disturbances such as low sodium, low potassium or low blood sugar can occur. These are all potentially life-threatening.
- A nasogastric tube can cause choking and extreme discomfort at placement and afterwards. At the time of insertion, it can be misplaced in the trachea and cause pneumonia. The tube can cause erosions and abrasions, even perforations (holes) in the nasal passages, esophagus, and stomach, and can cause acute and chronic bleeding. Aspiration pneumonia is a risk whenever an NG tube is in place. If a person is confused, he/she may need restraints to keep him/her from pulling the tube out. This can cause a whole host of problems, including psychic distress and increased agitation and anxiety, skin breakdown due to immobility, pneumonia due to immobility, and injury from restraints to name a few.
- A gastrostomy tube requires anesthesia during placement and has risks associated with the use of anesthesia. There is also a risk of infection of the abdominal wall and peritonitis (life threatening infection of the abdominal cavity). Gastrointestinal bleeding, blockage of the bowel or perforation of the bowel may occur. Diarrhea from the feeding formula is fairly common. Aspiration pneumonia is also common. If the person requires restraints to keep from pulling the tube out, the same complications listed above can occur.
- Intravenous fluids require IV tubing, with associated pain on insertion. Localized infection or cellulitis (a more serious infection of the skin that can spread) can occur. Thrombophlebitis (clotting in the vein) can occur and cause swelling and discomfort. Fluid overload is possible, causing swelling of the legs, arms, and body. Electrolyte imbalances such as low sodium or low potassium are common.

Are there any beneficial effects of dehydration?

Dehydration can actually have several potential benefits for a person who is at the end stages of his/her life:

- Secretions in the lungs are diminished, so cough and congestion are less, and procedure.
- Dehydration can lead to a melting away of the swelling and increased comfort in a person who has edema (swelling of the body caused by excess body fluids) or ascites (fluid in the abdominal cavity).
- With dehydration, there is less fluid in the gastrointestinal tract, which may decrease nausea, vomiting, bloating and regurgitation.
- A dehydrated person has less urine output, thus less need to go to the bathroom. The bed bound patient develops skin irritation when he/she develops incontinence. There is also less need to place a foley catheter in such a person. Foley catheters are irritating, can cause extremely painful bladder spasms, and are known to increase the risk of serious infections of the urinary tract and body.

Artificial nutrition and hydration is a medical treatment, with intended beneficial effects but many side effects and complications attached to its use. Decisions about its use need to be based on a dispassionate look at what, if any, benefits will occur, what side effects and burdens are likely to occur, and what the individuals' and families' goals are for the treatment.

When artificial nutrition and hydration is more likely to be burdensome than helpful, it should be avoided or discontinued. Nurturing can be expressed in more helpful ways, such as gentle presence, touch, talking with the person (regardless of his/her ability to respond), keeping the person's lips and mouth moist, gently massaging the skin using lubricants, praying with the person, or playing favorite music selections. These alternative ways of nurturing can be very powerful and moving for both the person with the life-threatening illness and his/her loved one.

The materials on this website are released under the Creative Commons Zero Waiver 1.0 (CC0). You may reproduce all or part of these materials as long as you cite American Hospice Foundation and link to this website (www.americanhospice.org).

What are some medical treatments that need to be understood when undertaking advance care planning?

By Cheryl Arenella, MD, MPH
American Hospice Foundation
www.americanhospice.org

Cardiopulmonary resuscitation (CPR)

What does it involve? A person whose heart has stopped, and who has stopped breathing, undergoes interventions to restart the heart and the breathing:

"Chemical Code"

What does it involve? Occasionally, a person will opt not to have mechanical resuscitation, but still desires the administration of medications intravenously to restart the heart, correct the heart rhythm, or support failing blood pressure.

Ventilator support

What does it involve? A person who is unable to breathe well enough to get a sufficient amount of oxygen to the body may need to have a tube inserted down the nose or throat, or surgically through the neck, into the trachea. This would then be connected to a ventilator (breathing machine), which would breathe for the patient.

Continuous Positive Airway Pressure (CPAP) and Bilevel Positive Airway Pressure (BiPAP)

What does it involve? The person who has difficulty breathing may use a mask over the nose only or over both nose and mouth, connected by tubes to a machine that delivers positive air pressure to the person's airways. This positive pressure helps keep the airways open and decreases the work of breathing for some patients.

Dialysis

What does it entail? If a person develops renal failure, toxins are not filtered out of the blood by the kidneys and build up in the body. A dialysis machine filters the toxins out of the blood. The person needs to have a way to take blood from the body, pass the blood through the machine, and return cleansed blood to the body. Usually, an internal connection from an artery to a vein is created surgically in the person's arm.

Total Parenteral Nutrition (TPN)

What does this involve? A person who is not able to take food by mouth, or who has a non-functioning gastrointestinal (GI) tract, may be given basic nutrients through a catheter (small tube) inserted into a vein. Often, the catheter is permanently or semi-permanently placed in a major vein.

Intravenous fluids (IV fluids)

What does this involve? A person who becomes dehydrated due to an inability to take enough fluids by mouth or an excessive loss of fluids through vomiting, diarrhea, or through the skin may have fluids replaced by having a catheter placed in the vein delivering solutions to the body.

Enteral tube placement

What does it entail? A tube may be placed either through the nose into the stomach or inserted surgically directly into the gastrointestinal tract through the abdominal wall. This tube may be used for administering food or medicine to the person, or it may be used to decompress the bowel if a bowel blockage is causing the buildup of air or gastrointestinal contents.

Surgery

What is involved? Depending on the type of surgery, surgical procedures can be more or less burdensome, have more or fewer complications, and be more or less debilitating.

Transfusions with blood and blood products

What is involved? The person who is anemic, or who has a deficiency of a certain type of blood product, can have blood or blood products transfused through a catheter placed in a vein. The person needs to be "typed and crossed" (i.e., the blood type must be checked for compatibility of the blood products he/she will receive), which requires having a blood sample drawn.

Use of antibiotics

What is involved? Antibiotics are given to fight infections in a person's body. They can be given by mouth or, for more severe infections, injected intramuscularly (into a muscle) or intravenously (into a vein).

Admission to the Intensive Care Unit (ICU)

What is involved? The intensive care unit is generally meant for a person who is reversibly critically ill who desires full resuscitation should cardiorespiratory arrest occur. This person will benefit from very invasive technology to reverse critical illness. Close monitoring of the patient, electronically and by medical personnel, is the norm.

Hospitalization

When should hospitalization be considered? Hospitals are useful for care of severely ill patients who have reversible conditions when the care cannot be managed in an outpatient setting.

Diagnostic tests

What is involved? Diagnostic tests may include blood tests, imaging tests (X-rays and scans), or invasive testing (e.g., looking into the esophagus, lung, stomach, or bowel with scopes and taking biopsies through the scopes).

What about implanted pacemakers and defibrillators?

These days, many people have had surgical placement of pacemakers to regulate the rate of the heart or implanted defibrillators that deliver a "shock" to the heart if it stops or goes into a dangerous rhythm. If a person with such an implanted device becomes terminally ill, and the goal is for comfort care only, the device can be turned off rather easily by the use of a magnet in close proximity to the device. A person can include instructions in his/her advance directive to turn off a pacemaker or a defibrillator at the appropriate time.

In addition to sorting through which treatments may not be desired, a person doing advance care planning should indicate what treatments he/she desires:

- Having skin care with body lotions
- Having routine moistening of mouth and eyes when drying occurs
- Having loved ones be able to visit at any time
- Having gentle massage and range of motion to prevent stiffness
- Having favored music played
- Etc.

A person should also give thought to whether or not he/she wishes to donate his or her body or organs or undergo an autopsy.

The materials on this website are released under the Creative Commons Zero Waiver 1.0 (CC0). You may reproduce all or part of these materials as long as you cite American Hospice Foundation and link to this website (www.americanhospice.org).

SECTION 4

CHAPTER 5

Corporate America and Alzheimer's

Impacting Corporate America

Harvard Business School Study

According to a recent study, businesses are pretty much oblivious to the number of employees who are caring for family members at home.

More than 80% of the employees surveyed said their caregiving duties impacted their work, yet less than 25% of employers felt that caregiving impacted the work of the very same employees.

The impact on corporate workforce is a problem and not only among lower-level employees. According to the Harvard report, the percentage of staff who left their jobs to care for a family member were:

- Senior leadership: 61%
- Manager of managers: 53%
- Manager of employees: 44%
- Employee: 23%

Also, interesting about this report is that more men (38%) than women (27%) said they quit to care for someone. The cost to replace and train new employees is enormous. For example, it can take months to hire a senior executive, and search firms charge between 20% and 30% of the first-year salary for a new candidate.

Caregivers: Rand Corporation

The Rand Corporation is an American nonprofit global policy think tank created in 1948. They have studied the financial cost of employee caregivers on American corporations.

The study estimates that three out of five family caregivers are in the labor force, and that these double-duty workers are providing 22 billion hours of unpaid care each year, saving money for our healthcare system, but costing these family caregivers billions of dollars annually in expenditures and lost wages. It is also estimates that American companies **lose** $25 billion annually due to the lost productivity of caregiver employees

Working caregivers report that their caregiving role impacts their careers in many ways. They feel torn between their work duties and their loved ones' needs, experiencing elevated stress both at work and at home. They often miss out on opportunities for advancement and promotion and must cut back on business travel and training. They use all their vacation time and sick days to provide care, sometimes taking unpaid leave as well. And if they quit their job to care for their loved one, they often find that they are unable to step back into a position comparable to their former level upon their return to the workforce. AARP also reports that 25 percent of today's retirees left the workforce earlier than they had planned to care for an ill spouse or parent.

Leaving the workforce early, taking a long leave from work, or turning down opportunities for advancement usually is a bad idea, financially speaking. It can have a major impact on lifetime earnings. Experts caution that people who sacrifice their paid work to care for an elder spouse, parent or other family member may find themselves, in turn, without adequate resources to fund their own retirement and long-term care due to loss of wages and Social Security earnings, and underfunded pensions or retirement accounts.

Employer Programs

Workers aren't the only ones impacted by elder care. Companies are learning that caregiver support programs make a big difference by raising productivity, building employee loyalty, and cutting down on the cost of turnover and training. Find out if your company offers family leave, flex time, telecommuting, job sharing, or an employee assistance and wellness program with resources for caregivers. Though some caregivers hesitate to discuss their situation with the boss, not wanting to bring personal problems to work, it's usually best to explain what is going on, and to express your continuous commitment to your job.

SECTION 5

CHAPTER 6

TIPS

Tips for the Caregiver

Working at various memory care centers as a volunteer gave me the opportunity to meet and observe many family members caring for their loved one. It also allowed me to see firsthand the quality of care and the methods used to manage fifty or more very needy patients on a daily basis. Certified Nursing Assistants (CNAs) are the front line of the caring effort. These are also the aides who are on call for many home care dementia patients. As with any group, some are more proficient than others.

Tip #1
Classes
Caring for a dementia patient is a long-term ordeal. Some illnesses last five to ten years or more. Therefore, it might be wise for a family member to consider taking the CNA training course. Every state offers different programs that generally last from one to two months with much of it being online.

Tip #2
Communications :
- Refrain from correcting the person when they're telling a story incorrectly or repeatedly asking the same questions.
- Use a positive tone of voice since people with dementia are susceptible to your frustration or anger.
- If your loved one is resisting something you want them to do, such as bathe, wait and try again later. People with dementia can be very sensitive to water and room temperature.
- Research shows that response time for a person with dementia can be delayed by up to thirty seconds. For you as a caregiver, this delay might be frustrating. It's also easy to misinterpret a delay as the person's inability to comprehend your message.
- Use visual demonstrations and tactile or hands-on cues to illustrate your words.

- Brush your hair and brush teeth together.
- If your senior refuses or complains about taking medication, try taking your medication at the same time.
- Be patient, supportive, and friendly. At every stage of dementia, there is a person behind the patient. Listen with your ears, eyes, and heart.
- When the going gets tough, distract and redirect.
- Keep it simple. Treat the person with dignity and respect.
- Avoid talking down to the person or as if he or she isn't there.
- Ask yes or no questions.
- Approach from the front. Always try to approach a person with dementia from the front, so he or she has an opportunity to recognize you. Keep in mind too that in the later stages of dementia, the person's range of vision may become more limited, so you may need to make further adaptations.

Tip #3

Simple but important:

- Use a fixed routine. Eat, shower, sleep, etc. at specific times.
- Be aware of medication interaction or urinary tract infections, which can lead to symptoms getting worse.
- Focus on hydration. As people age, they lose their thirst mechanism, and dehydration can have serious consequences.
- Create good sleeping habits by limiting naps and caffeine.
- Make sure the bathroom is warm.
- Install grab bars to reduce the fear of falling.
- Get a shower chair and a handheld sprayer.
- Use a towel to cover your senior's shoulders (and lap if using a shower chair) to keep them warm and maintain as much privacy as possible.
- Keep the door to the bathroom open so your senior can see the toilet or put a sign on the door.
- Keep the light on in the bathroom all the time.
- Carry extra clothes, supplies for clean-up, and a plastic bag whenever you take your senior out.

Tip #4

Dealing with the Silence:

The normal daily chat about the weather, current events, and family issues wind down and eventually cease when your loved one suffers from Alzheimer's disease. This is a terrible burden for the family caregiver. One solution to keep some level of mutual interest is to make a "personal play list" of whatever they enjoyed in the past on an iPad or computer.

For instance, if their hobby was tennis, soccer, golf, car racing, music, or just watching animals play - YouTube has it. Go to YouTube.com and type in your request. You will see many options to choose from and click on the one that best suits your loved one.

It's best to choose the highlights to eliminate non-action delays. For example: just use the Wimbledon Match highlights; the 2021 Masters Tournament highlights; the Indianapolis 500; or soccer greats like Pelé, Christiano Ronaldo, and Lionel Messi highlights and not the entire game or event.

List their favorite songs, artists, and TV series they enjoyed when younger. One with almost universal appeal is Andre Rieu's concerts because they contain music and dancing. One of the most appealing forms of entertainment is simply watching animal videos.

Tip #5

Smart 911

Saves Time and Saves Lives

Smart 911 is available in many communities. On your computer search for SMART 911. The site provides all the necessary demographic and medical information relevant to you and your loved one. There is even a place to list identifying features and photos in case your patient wanders from home. When you call 911 let the dispatcher know you are listed on SMART 911 and they can access all this important data. Smart 911 is a national service meaning your Smart 911 Safety Profile travels with you and is visible to any participating 911 center nationwide.

Tip #6

The Alzheimer's Store

Over 300 items are available on this website to assist in caregiving.

The great selection features objects from anti-scalding devices, confounding door locks, color-coded picture phones, refrigerator latches, commode accommodations, stove fire alerts, gifts, and so much more.

www.alzstore.com

Tip #7

Travel Tips

Identification: Make sure that all travel documents and identification are readily accessible. It may be helpful for the person to wear a document holder.

Timing: Travel during the time of day that is best for the person. For example, if he or she becomes tired or more agitated in the late afternoon, avoid traveling at this time.

Meals: Stay as close to your normal routine as possible. For example, keep mealtimes and bedtimes on a similar schedule. Eating in a home may be a better choice than at a crowded restaurant.

Change: Environmental changes can trigger wandering or confusion. Consider enrolling in a wandering response service. The nationwide emergency response service facilitates the safe return of individuals living with Alzheimer's disease or other dementias who may wander or have a medical emergency.

Plan: Carry with you an itinerary that includes details about each destination. Give copies to family members or friends you will be visiting or to emergency contacts at home. Carry plenty of hand wipes for any spills.

Air Travel: Allow for plenty of time. Two caregivers should be present for plane travel. Try to fly on direct flights only to avoid layovers. Preboard the aircraft. Pack all medications in a carry-on bag (do not put them in the checked luggage). Contact TSA to determine if a pass can be issued to the caregivers to escort the passenger through security to the gate.

Driving: If an Alzheimer's patient becomes agitated or nervous, pull over. Do not try to calm them while driving. Be aware they may attempt to leave a moving car.

Limitations: Be realistic! Assess the limitations of the Alzheimer's person and your own. Can you handle them if they become agitated, disoriented, aggressive, paranoid, etc.? Discuss increasing medications for the trip with your doctor.

Hotels/Motels: Call ahead to advise staff of your specific needs so they can be prepared to assist you. Request a quiet room, avoid sliding glass doors, bring a door alarm or a childproof doorknob cover.

Alzheimer's Disease

Packing: Pack necessary medications, up-to-date medical information, a list of emergency contacts, and photocopies of important legal documents.

Have a backup plan: Be prepared to react to any mishaps without becoming overly anxious.

Tip #8

A Safer Bathroom

Install a commode chair for safety.

Install grab bars in the shower or tub.

A handheld shower head makes it easier to bathe while sitting.

The illustration below shows a shower padded commode chair with wheels.

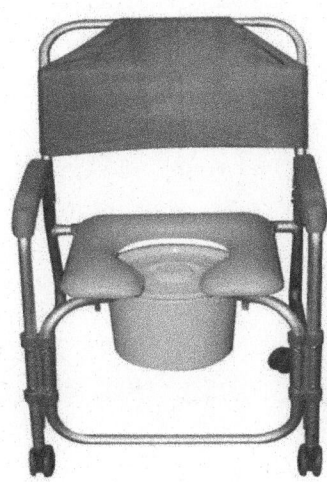

Tip #9

Support Groups

Support Groups are an inexpensive and effective way to assist people dealing with Alzheimer's care. Small groups of people gather to share common problems and experiences. People have the opportunity to discuss what they are going through and share the practical insights that can only come from firsthand experience.

For Support Group Information:

Google: Mental Health America's Support Group Facilitation Guide

Tip #10

Other Considerations - End of Life Wishes

Start the process early when the disease is diagnosed and before the confusion begins. Answers can be revised as circumstances change.

- Do you want to spend your last days at home, a hospital, or a nursing home?
- Do you want extended treatments, or will you accept palliative care if recommended by a doctor?
- Which family member will be your decision maker?
- Are there treatments you would want (or not want), such as feeding tubes or heart resuscitation?
- I would like to leave my special items, such as jewelry, clothing, etc. to _____
- The safe deposit box key for XYZ bank is kept_____?
- What credit cards should be cancelled?
- I leave my car to_____
- I want my obituary to say_____
- I want to be buried_____
- I want to be cremated
- I want a military funeral
- I want these friends and family members to be notified.
- My passwords & usernames for access to electronic devices are_____
- My brokerage account number is_____
- My broker is_____
- My banker is_____
- Check my employer benefit programs
- My deeds and titles are located_____
- I have other assets_____
- Contact Social Security
- Contact the VA
- Notify my creditors_____
- Discontinue my subscriptions, cable, cellphone, internet_____
- Notify the Utility company_____
- Forward my mail
- File my last tax return
- I would like to leave my pet to_____.

SECTION 6

CHAPTER 7

Resources

Helpful Resources for You and Your Family

The Alzheimer's Association

The leading health organization in Alzheimer's care, support, and research. The mission is to eliminate Alzheimer's disease through the advancement of research; to provide and enhance care and support for all affected; and to reduce the risk of dementia through the promotion of brain health.

Website: alz.org

The Fisher Center for Alzheimer's Research Foundation

This organization provides millions of dollars for novel Alzheimer's research primarily conducted by the late Nobel Prize laureate Dr. Paul Greengard and his team of over sixty internationally renowned scientists at the Fisher Center lab at the Rockefeller University, plus other leading research institutes around the world.

The Fisher Center lab at the Rockefeller University is one of the largest and most modern scientific facilities in the world dedicated to solving the puzzle of Alzheimer's disease.

Website: alzinfo.org

The National Institutes of Health (NIH)

A part of the US Department of Health and Human Services, NIH is the nation's medical research agency—making important discoveries that improve health and save lives. It is made up of twenty-seven different components called institutes and centers. Each has its own specific research agenda, often focusing on specific diseases or body systems.

Website: nih.gov   https://www.nia.nih.gov/alzheimers/topics/alzheimers-basics

Johns Hopkins Memory and Alzheimer's Treatment Center

One of the things that sets this memory center apart is the support they provide to both patients and families not only in the form of individual care but also with a monthly social club, books, web links, podcasts, an advisory council, and a family resource center.

https://www.hopkinsmedicine.org/psychiatry/specialtyareas/memorycenter.

Centers for Disease Control and Prevention (CDC)

The CDC targets their research to the largest health problems that cause death and disability for Americans.

Source: cdc.gov

BrightFocus Foundation

BrightFocus funds exceptional scientific research worldwide to defeat Alzheimer's disease, macular degeneration, and glaucoma, providing expert information on these heartbreaking diseases.

Source: brightfocus.org

Byrd Alzheimer's Center and Research Institute

The University of South Florida Health Byrd Alzheimer's Center and Research Institute is dedicated to the prevention, treatment, and cure of Alzheimer's disease and related disorders.

The institution is a multidisciplinary center of excellence at the University of South Florida that provides compassionate family centered patient care, performs cutting edge research, and delivers quality public and professional education, doctors, clinicians, and educators. The institute is at the forefront of Alzheimer's research and care.

Source: health.usf.edu

The Cleveland Clinic

WEBINAR SERIES:

A virtual online informational session hosted by the Cleveland Alzheimer's Disease Research Center aiming to provide timely information and brain-healthy activities by area professionals.

Source: clevelandclinc.org

Support Groups

Support programs provide education and information to dementia caregivers looking for suggestions on ways to cope with anxiety, depression, and other mental health issues. These programs also help caregivers alleviate stress while providing a sense of dignity and independence to the person with Alzheimer's Disease.Source: alz.org

All the above nonprofit organizations need and appreciate your financial support.

Much of the material in this booklet is available on various government agency websites for no charge. Many of these government websites on-line publications continually update as the agency learns more about a specific disease or condition. Therefore, check for updates to ensure the latest information being offered to users.

References

Alzheimer's Association. "2020 Alzheimer's disease facts and figures." Accessed 3/12/2022. (https://alz-journals.onlinelibrary.wiley.com/doi/full/10.1002/alz.12068).

Alzheimer's Association. "Stages of Alzheimer's." Accessed 3/12/2022. (https://www.alz.org/alzheimers-dementia/stages).

Alzheimer's Association. "What is Dementia?" Accessed 3/12/2022. (https://www.alz.org/alzheimers-dementia/what-is-dementia).

American Academy of Neurology. Brain&Life. "Dementia 101: Know the Different Types of Dementia. Accessed 3/15/2022." (https://www.brainandlife.org/articles/not-all-dementia-is-alzheimers-disease-knowing-the-difference-affects/).

Centers for Disease Control and Prevention. "Alzheimer's Disease and Healthy Aging: What is Dementia?" Accessed 3/12/2022. (https://www.cdc.gov/aging/dementia/index.html).

Centers for Disease Control and Prevention. "U.S. burden of Alzheimer's disease, related dementias to double by 2060." Accessed 3/12/2022. (https://www.cdc.gov/media/releases/2018/p0920-alzheimers-burden-double-2060.html).

Centers for Disease Control and Prevention. "What is Dementia?" Accessed 3/12/2022. (https://www.cdc.gov/aging/dementia/index.html).

Family Caregiver Alliance. National Center on Caregiving. "Is this Dementia and What Does it Mean?" Accessed 3/12/2022. (https://www.caregiver.org/resource/is-this-dementia-what-does-it-mean/).

Mace, Nancy L. and Peter Rabins. *Understanding Dementia Diseases /Types of Dementia Diseases The 36-Hour Day*. Sixth edition. Baltimore, MD: John Hopkins University Press, 2017.

National Institute of Neurological Disorders & Stroke. "Dementia Information Page." Accessed 3/12/2022. (https://www.ninds.nih.gov/Disorders/All-Disorders/Dementia-Information-Page).

National Institute on Aging. "Do Memory Problems Always Mean Alzheimer's Disease?" Accessed 3/12/2022. (https://www.nia.nih.gov/health/do-memory-problems-always-mean-alzheimers-disease).

National Institute on Aging. "What is Dementia?: Symptoms, Types, and Diagnosis." Accessed 3/12/2022. (https://www.nia.nih.gov/health/what-dementia-symptoms-types-and-diagnosis).

NHS Choices. "Dementia Guide." Accessed 3/12/2022. (https://www.nhs.uk/conditions/dementia/about/).

Reisberg, Barry and Emile H. Franssen. "Clinical stages of Alzheimer's disease." In *The Encyclopedia of Visual Medicine Series: An Atlas of Alzheimer's Disease*, pages 12-20. Pearl River, NY: Parthenon, 1999.

Robinson, L. "Dementia: Timely diagnosis and early intervention." *BMJ*. 2015; 350:h3029. Accessed 3/12/2022. (https://www.bmj.com/content/350/bmj.h3029).

Sheen, Bishop Fulton J. *The World's First Love: Mary, Mother of God*. San Francisco: Ignatius Press, 2010.

APPENDIX A

Helpful Worksheets

(Permission is granted to make copies of the following pages.)

MEDICATIONS FOR
_____

Physician: _____
Pharmacist: _____

MEDICATION	DOSE/MG	MORNING	LUNCH	BEDTIME
_____	_____	_____	_____	_____
_____	_____	_____	_____	_____
_____	_____	_____	_____	_____
_____	_____	_____	_____	_____
_____	_____	_____	_____	_____
_____	_____	_____	_____	_____
_____	_____	_____	_____	_____
_____	_____	_____	_____	_____
_____	_____	_____	_____	_____

QUESTIONS FOR MY DOCTOR:

NOTES:

APPENDIX B

THE STORY OF OUR LADY OF FATIMA

<u>Fatima</u>, a small community in central Portugal is a location and the name of a major event in history.

The "Miracle at Fatima" is arguably the most well-known apparition of the Blessed Mother. Her appearance to three shepherd children in Portugal in 1917 was, according to many witnesses, accompanied by several unexplained events, including a shared vision of the sun dancing and moving about erratically in the sky.

It is a story of three shepherd children who in 1917 claimed they saw the Virgin Mary, Mother of God in the fields outside the small city. The children claimed to have seen the Marian apparition on six occasions and stated that the last one would be October 13, 1917. An estimated 70,000 pilgrims went to the site for the last prophesied apparition. Some of them reported what has been referred to as the Miracle of the Sun.

On that day, one of the spectators, a professor, shared his experience and what he saw:

"It must have been 1:30 p.m when there arose, at the exact spot where the children were, a column of smoke, thin, fine and bluish, which extended up to perhaps two meters above their heads, and evaporated at that height. This phenomenon, perfectly visible to the naked eye, lasted for a few seconds. Not having noted how long it had lasted, I cannot say whether it was more or less than a minute. The smoke dissipated abruptly, and after some time, it came back to occur a second time, then a third time

"The sky, which had been overcast all day, suddenly cleared; the rain stopped and it looked as if the sun were about to fill with light the countryside that the wintery morning had made so gloomy. I was looking at the spot of the apparitions in a serene, if cold, expectation of something happening and with diminishing curiosity because a long time had passed without anything to excite my attention. The sun, a few moments before, had broken through the thick layer of clouds which hid it and now shone clearly and intensely.

"Suddenly I heard the uproar of thousands of voices, and I saw the whole multitude spread out in that vast space at my feet…turn their backs to that spot where, until then, all their expectations had been focused, and look at the sun on the other side. I turned around, too, toward the point commanding their gaze and I could see the sun, like a very clear disc, with its sharp edge, which gleamed without hurting the sight. It could not be confused with the sun seen through a fog (there was no fog at that moment), for it was neither veiled nor dim. At Fatima, it kept its light and heat, and stood out clearly in the sky, with a sharp edge, like a large gaming table. The most astonishing thing was to be able to stare at the solar disc for a long time, brilliant with light and heat, without hurting the eyes or damaging the retina. [During this time], the sun's disc did not remain immobile, it had a giddy motion, [but] not like the twinkling of a star in all its brilliance for it spun round upon itself in a mad whirl.

Alzheimer's Disease

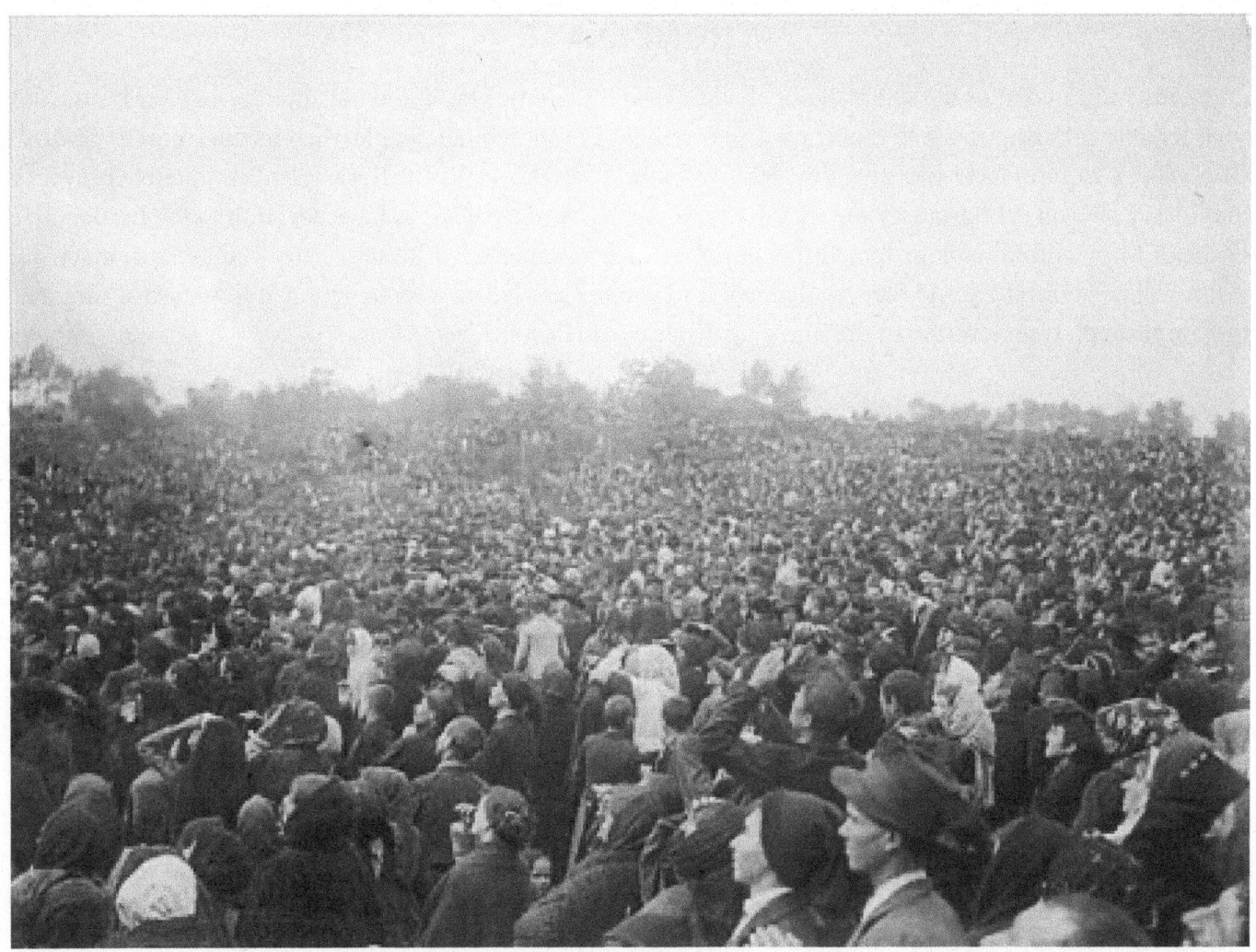

"During the solar phenomenon, which I have just described, there were also changes of color in the atmosphere. Looking at the sun, I noticed that everything was becoming darkened. I looked first at the nearest objects and then extended my glance further afield as far as the horizon. I saw everything had assumed an amethyst color. Objects around me, the sky and the atmosphere, were of the same color. Everything both near and far had changed, taking on the color of old yellow damask. People looked as if they were suffering from jaundice, and I recall a sensation of amusement at seeing them look so ugly and unattractive. My own hand was the same color.

"Then, suddenly, one heard a clamor, a cry of anguish breaking from all the people. The sun, whirling wildly, seemed all at once to loosen itself from the firmament and, blood red, advance threateningly upon the earth as if to crush us with its huge and fiery weight. The sensation during those moments was truly terrible.

"All the phenomena which I have described were observed by me in a calm and serene state of mind without any emotional disturbance. It is for others to interpret and explain them. Finally, I must declare that never, before or after October 13 [1917], have I observed similar atmospheric or solar phenomena."

THE MESSAGE:

Our Lady indicated to us the specific root of all the troubles in the world, the one that causes world wars and such terrible suffering: sin. She then gave a solution, first to individual people, then to the Church's leaders. God asks each one of us to stop offending Him. We must pray, especially the Rosary. By this frequent prayer of the Rosary, we will get the graces we need to overcome sin. God wants us to have devotion to the Immaculate Heart of Mary and to work to spread this devotion throughout the world. Our Lady said, "My Immaculate Heart will be your refuge and the way that will lead you to God." If we wish to go to God, we have a sure way to Him through true devotion to the Immaculate Heart of His Mother.